This report contains the collective views of an internatio
experts and does not necessarily represent the decisions
of the United Nations Environment Programme, the Inte............. ......
Organization or the World Health Organization.

Environmental Health Criteria 225

PRINCIPLES FOR EVALUATING HEALTH RISKS TO REPRODUCTION ASSOCIATED WITH EXPOSURE TO CHEMICALS

Initial drafts prepared by Dr P. Foster, Research Triangle Park, NC, USA; Dr W. Foster, Los Angeles, CA, USA; Dr C. Hughes, Los Angeles, CA, USA; Dr C. Kimmel, Washington, DC, USA; Dr S. Selevan, Washington, DC, USA; Dr N. Skakkebaek, Copenhagen, Denmark; Dr F. Sullivan, Brighton, England; Dr S. Tabacova, Sofia, Bulgaria; Dr J. Toppari, Turku, Finland; and Dr B. Ulbrich, Berlin, Germany

Published under the joint sponsorship of the United Nations Environment Programme, the International Labour Organization and the World Health Organization, and produced within the framework of the Inter-Organization Programme for the Sound Management of Chemicals.

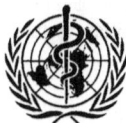

World Health Organization
Geneva, 2001

The **International Programme on Chemical Safety (IPCS)**, established in 1980, is a joint venture of the United Nations Environment Programme (UNEP), the International Labour Organization (ILO) and the World Health Organization (WHO). The overall objectives of the IPCS are to establish the scientific basis for assessment of the risk to human health and the environment from exposure to chemicals, through international peer review processes, as a prerequisite for the promotion of chemical safety, and to provide technical assistance in strengthening national capacities for the sound management of chemicals.

The **Inter-Organization Programme for the Sound Management of Chemicals (IOMC)** was established in 1995 by UNEP, ILO, the Food and Agriculture Organization of the United Nations, WHO, the United Nations Industrial Development Organization, the United Nations Institute for Training and Research and the Organisation for Economic Co-operation and Development (Participating Organizations), following recommendations made by the 1992 UN Conference on Environment and Development to strengthen cooperation and increase coordination in the field of chemical safety. The purpose of the IOMC is to promote coordination of the policies and activities pursued by the Participating Organizations, jointly or separately, to achieve the sound management of chemicals in relation to human health and the environment.

WHO Library Cataloguing-in-Publication Data

Principles for evaluating health risks to reproduction associated with exposure to chemicals.

(Environmental health criteria ; 225)

1.Reproduction - physiology 2.Reproduction - drug effects
3.Fertility - drug effects 4.Fetal development - drug effects
5.Environmental exposure 6.Risk assessment I.International Programme for Chemical Safety II.Series

ISBN 92 4 157225 6   (NLM classification: QZ 59)
ISSN 0250-863X

Printed in Finland
2001/13946 – Vammala – 5000

CONTENTS

ENVIRONMENTAL HEALTH CRITERIA FOR PRINCIPLES FOR EVALUATING HEALTH RISKS TO REPRODUCTION ASSOCIATED WITH EXPOSURE TO CHEMICALS

NOTE TO READERS OF THE CRITERIA MONOGRAPHS

Every effort has been made to present information in the criteria monographs as accurately as possible without unduly delaying their publication. In the interest of all users of the Environmental Health Criteria monographs, readers are requested to communicate any errors that may have occurred to the Director of the International Programme on Chemical Safety, World Health Organization, Geneva, Switzerland, in order that they may be included in corrigenda.

* * *

A detailed data profile and a legal file can be obtained from the International Register of Potentially Toxic Chemicals, Case postale 356, 1219 Châtelaine, Geneva, Switzerland (telephone no. + 41 22 – 9799111, fax no. + 41 22 – 7973460, E-mail irptc@unep.ch).

Environmental Health Criteria

PREAMBLE

Objectives

In 1973, the WHO Environmental Health Criteria Programme was initiated with the following objectives:

(i)   to assess information on the relationship between exposure to environmental pollutants and human health, and to provide guidelines for setting exposure limits;

(ii) to identify new or potential pollutants;

(iii) to identify gaps in knowledge concerning the health effects of pollutants;

(iv) to promote the harmonization of toxicological and epidemiological methods in order to have internationally comparable results.

The first Environmental Health Criteria (EHC) monograph, on mercury, was published in 1976, and since that time an ever-increasing number of assessments of chemicals and of physical effects have been produced. In addition, many EHC monographs have been devoted to evaluating toxicological methodology, e.g., for genetic, neurotoxic, teratogenic and nephrotoxic effects. Other publications have been concerned with epidemiological guidelines, evaluation of short-term tests for carcinogens, biomarkers, effects on the elderly and so forth.

Since its inauguration, the EHC Programme has widened its scope, and the importance of environmental effects, in addition to health effects, has been increasingly emphasized in the total evaluation of chemicals.

The original impetus for the Programme came from World Health Assembly resolutions and the recommendations of the 1972 UN Conference on the Human Environment. Subsequently, the work became an integral part of the International Programme on Chemical

Safety (IPCS), a cooperative programme of UNEP, ILO and WHO. In this manner, with the strong support of the new partners, the importance of occupational health and environmental effects was fully recognized. The EHC monographs have become widely established, used and recognized throughout the world.

The recommendations of the 1992 UN Conference on Environment and Development and the subsequent establishment of the Intergovernmental Forum on Chemical Safety with the priorities for action in the six programme areas of Chapter 19, Agenda 21, all lend further weight to the need for EHC assessments of the risks of chemicals.

Scope

The criteria monographs are intended to provide critical reviews on the effects on human health and the environment of chemicals and of combinations of chemicals and physical and biological agents. As such, they include and review studies that are of direct relevance for the evaluation. However, they do not describe *every* study carried out. Worldwide data are used and are quoted from original studies, not from abstracts or reviews. Both published and unpublished reports are considered, and it is incumbent on the authors to assess all the articles cited in the references. Preference is always given to published data. Unpublished data are used only when relevant published data are absent or when they are pivotal to the risk assessment. A detailed policy statement is available that describes the procedures used for unpublished proprietary data so that this information can be used in the evaluation without compromising its confidential nature (WHO (1990) Revised Guidelines for the Preparation of Environmental Health Criteria Monographs. PCS/90.69, Geneva, World Health Organization).

In the evaluation of human health risks, sound human data, whenever available, are preferred to animal data. Animal and *in vitro* studies provide support and are used mainly to supply evidence missing from human studies. It is mandatory that research on human subjects is conducted in full accord with ethical principles, including the provisions of the Helsinki Declaration.

The EHC monographs are intended to assist national and international authorities in making risk assessments and subsequent risk management decisions. They represent a thorough evaluation of risks and are not, in any sense, recommendations for regulation or standard setting. These latter are the exclusive purview of national and regional governments.

Content

The layout of EHC monographs for chemicals is outlined below.

- Summary — a review of the salient facts and the risk evaluation of the chemical
- Identity — physical and chemical properties, analytical methods
- Sources of exposure
- Environmental transport, distribution and transformation
- Environmental levels and human exposure
- Kinetics and metabolism in laboratory animals and humans
- Effects on laboratory mammals and *in vitro* test systems
- Effects on humans
- Effects on other organisms in the laboratory and field
- Evaluation of human health risks and effects on the environment
- Conclusions and recommendations for protection of human health and the environment
- Further research
- Previous evaluations by international bodies, e.g., IARC, JECFA, JMPR

Selection of chemicals

Since the inception of the EHC Programme, the IPCS has organized meetings of scientists to establish lists of priority chemicals for subsequent evaluation. Such meetings have been held in: Ispra, Italy, 1980; Oxford, United Kingdom, 1984; Berlin, Germany, 1987; and North Carolina, USA, 1995. The selection of chemicals has been based on the following criteria: the existence of scientific evidence that the substance presents a hazard to human health and/or the environment; the possible use, persistence, accumulation or degradation of the substance shows that there may be significant human or environmental exposure; the size and nature of populations at risk (both human and other species) and risks for the environment; international concern, i.e., the substance is of major interest to several countries; adequate data on the hazards are available.

If an EHC monograph is proposed for a chemical not on the priority list, the IPCS Secretariat consults with the cooperating organizations and all the Participating Institutions before embarking on the preparation of the monograph.

Procedures

The order of procedures that result in the publication of an EHC monograph is shown in the flow chart on the next page. A designated staff member of IPCS, responsible for the scientific quality of the document, serves as Responsible Officer (RO). The IPCS Editor is responsible for layout and language. The first draft, prepared by consultants or, more usually, staff from an IPCS Participating Institution, is based initially on data provided from the International Register of Potentially Toxic Chemicals and from reference databases such as Medline and Toxline.

The draft document, when received by the RO, may require an initial review by a small panel of experts to determine its scientific quality and objectivity. Once the RO finds the document acceptable as a first draft, it is distributed, in its unedited form, to well over 150 EHC contact points throughout the world who are asked to comment on its completeness and accuracy and, where necessary, provide additional material. The contact points, usually designated by governments, may be Participating Institutions, IPCS Focal Points or individual scientists known for their particular expertise. Generally, some four months are allowed before the comments are considered by the RO and author(s). A second draft incorporating comments received and approved by the Director, IPCS, is then distributed to Task Group members, who carry out the peer review, at least six weeks before their meeting.

The Task Group members serve as individual scientists, not as representatives of any organization, government or industry. Their function is to evaluate the accuracy, significance and relevance of the information in the document and to assess the health and environmental risks from exposure to the chemical. A summary and recommendations

EHC PREPARATION FLOW CHART

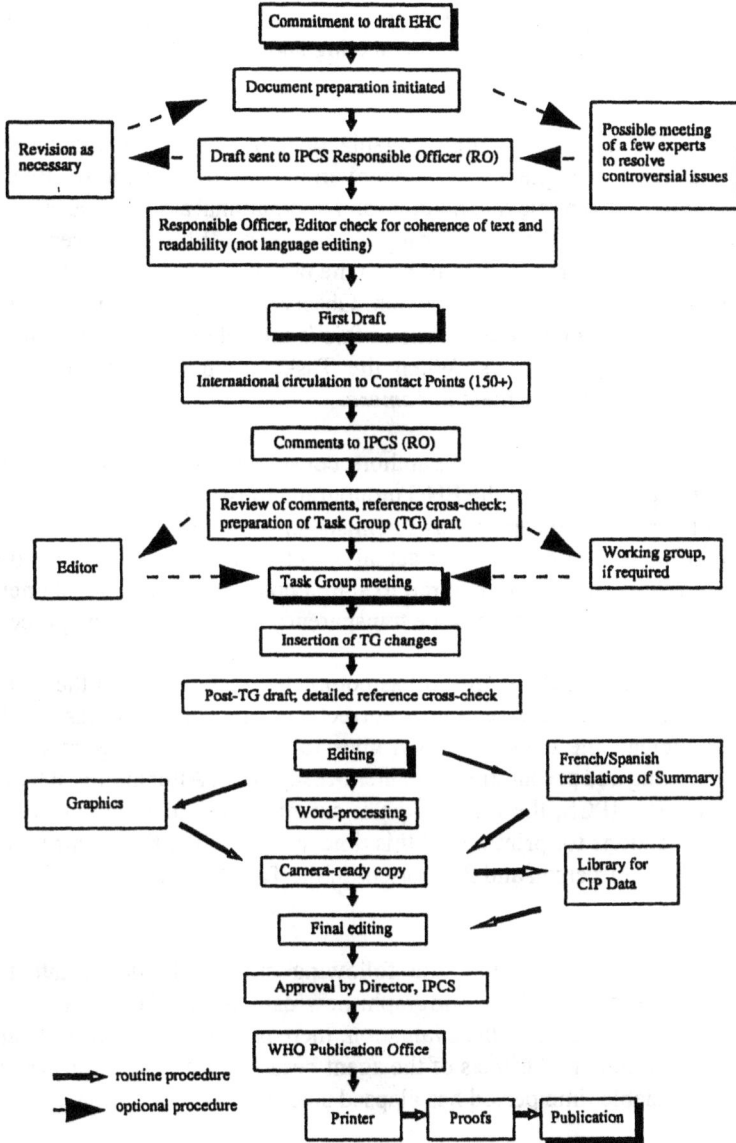

```
                         ┌─────────────────────────┐
                         │  Commitment to draft EHC │
                         └─────────────────────────┘
                                     │
                                     ▼
                         ┌─────────────────────────┐
                         │ Document preparation initiated │
                         └─────────────────────────┘
                                     │
┌──────────────┐        ┌─────────────────────────────────┐        ┌──────────────────────┐
│ Revision as  │ ◄───── │ Draft sent to IPCS Responsible Officer (RO) │ ◄──── │ Possible meeting      │
│ necessary    │        └─────────────────────────────────┘        │ of a few experts      │
└──────────────┘                    │                              │ to resolve            │
                                     ▼                              │ controversial issues  │
                 ┌──────────────────────────────────────────────┐  └──────────────────────┘
                 │ Responsible Officer, Editor check for coherence of text and │
                 │ readability (not language editing)            │
                 └──────────────────────────────────────────────┘
                                     │
                                     ▼
                         ┌─────────────────────────┐
                         │       First Draft       │
                         └─────────────────────────┘
                                     │
                                     ▼
                 ┌──────────────────────────────────────────────┐
                 │ International circulation to Contact Points (150+) │
                 └──────────────────────────────────────────────┘
                                     │
                                     ▼
                         ┌─────────────────────────┐
                         │  Comments to IPCS (RO)  │
                         └─────────────────────────┘
                                     │
                                     ▼
                 ┌──────────────────────────────────────────────┐
                 │ Review of comments, reference cross-check;    │
                 │ preparation of Task Group (TG) draft          │
                 └──────────────────────────────────────────────┘
┌──────────────┐                    │                              ┌──────────────────────┐
│   Editor     │ ─ ─ ─► ┌─────────────────────────┐ ◄─ ─ ─ ─ ─── │ Working group,        │
└──────────────┘        │   Task Group meeting     │              │ if required           │
                        └─────────────────────────┘              └──────────────────────┘
                                     │
                                     ▼
                         ┌─────────────────────────┐
                         │ Insertion of TG changes │
                         └─────────────────────────┘
                                     │
                                     ▼
                 ┌──────────────────────────────────────────────┐
                 │ Post-TG draft; detailed reference cross-check │
                 └──────────────────────────────────────────────┘
                                     │
                                     ▼
                         ┌─────────────────────────┐         ┌──────────────────────────┐
                         │        Editing          │ ──────► │ French/Spanish            │
                         └─────────────────────────┘         │ translations of Summary   │
                                     │                        └──────────────────────────┘
┌──────────────┐                    ▼
│  Graphics    │ ◄───── ┌─────────────────────────┐
└──────────────┘        │     Word-processing      │
                        └─────────────────────────┘
                                     │
                                     ▼
                         ┌─────────────────────────┐         ┌──────────────────────┐
                         │    Camera-ready copy     │ ──────► │ Library for           │
                         └─────────────────────────┘         │ CIP Data              │
                                     │                        └──────────────────────┘
                                     ▼
                         ┌─────────────────────────┐
                         │      Final editing      │
                         └─────────────────────────┘
                                     │
                                     ▼
                         ┌─────────────────────────┐
                         │ Approval by Director, IPCS │
                         └─────────────────────────┘
                                     │
                                     ▼
                         ┌─────────────────────────┐
                         │  WHO Publication Office  │
                         └─────────────────────────┘
                                     │
                                     ▼
   ───►  routine procedure
   ──►   optional procedure       ┌─────────┐   ┌────────┐   ┌─────────────┐
                                   │ Printer │──►│ Proofs │──►│ Publication │
                                   └─────────┘   └────────┘   └─────────────┘
```

for further research and improved safety aspects are also required. The composition of the Task Group is dictated by the range of expertise required for the subject of the meeting and by the need for a balanced geographical distribution.

The three cooperating organizations of the IPCS recognize the important role played by nongovernmental organizations. Representatives from relevant national and international associations may be invited to join the Task Group as observers. While observers may provide a valuable contribution to the process, they can speak only at the invitation of the Chairperson. Observers do not participate in the final evaluation of the chemical; this is the sole responsibility of the Task Group members. When the Task Group considers it to be appropriate, it may meet *in camera*.

All individuals who as authors, consultants or advisers participate in the preparation of the EHC monograph must, in addition to serving in their personal capacity as scientists, inform the RO if at any time a conflict of interest, whether actual or potential, could be perceived in their work. They are required to sign a conflict of interest statement. Such a procedure ensures the transparency and probity of the process.

When the Task Group has completed its review and the RO is satisfied as to the scientific correctness and completeness of the document, the document then goes for language editing, reference checking and preparation of camera-ready copy. After approval by the Director, IPCS, the monograph is submitted to the WHO Office of Publications for printing. At this time, a copy of the final draft is sent to the Chairperson and Rapporteur of the Task Group to check for any errors.

It is accepted that the following criteria should initiate the updating of an EHC monograph: new data are available that would substantially change the evaluation; there is public concern for health or environmental effects of the agent because of greater exposure; an appreciable time period has elapsed since the last evaluation.

All Participating Institutions are informed, through the EHC progress report, of the authors and institutions proposed for the drafting of the documents. A comprehensive file of all comments received on drafts of each EHC monograph is maintained and is available on request. The Chairpersons of Task Groups are briefed before each meeting on their role and responsibility in ensuring that these rules are followed.

WHO TASK GROUP ON ENVIRONMENTAL HEALTH CRITERIA FOR PRINCIPLES FOR EVALUATING HEALTH RISKS TO REPRODUCTION ASSOCIATED WITH EXPOSURE TO CHEMICALS

Members

Dr D. Anderson, TNO BIBRA Toxicology International Ltd., Surrey, United Kingdom

Prof. Dr E. Bustos-Obregón, University of Chile Medical School, Santiago, Chile

Prof. Dr I. Chahoud, Institut für Klinische Pharmakologie und Toxicologie, Berlin, Germany

Dr G. Daston, Procter & Gamble, Cincinnati, Ohio, USA

Dr P. Foster, Chemical Industry Institute of Toxicology, Research Triangle Park, North Carolina, USA

Dr W. Foster, Cedars-Sinai Medical Center, Los Angeles, California, USA

Dr U. Hass (representing Organisation for Economic Co-operation and Development), Soborg, Denmark

Dr C. Kimmel, US Environmental Protection Agency, Washington, DC, USA

Dr R. Little, National Institute of Environmental Health Sciences, Research Triangle Park, North Carolina, USA

Dr S. Selevan, US Environmental Protection Agency, Washington, DC, USA

Dr S. Tabacova, National Centre of Hygiene, Medical Ecology and Hygiene, Sofia, Bulgaria

Dr J. Toppari, University of Turku, Turku, Finland

Dr B. Ulbrich, Institute for Drugs and Medical Devices, Berlin, Germany

Dr M. Yasuda, Hiroshima School of Medicine, Hiroshima, Japan

Secretariat

Dr B.-H. Chen, Shanghai, China

Dr T. Damstra, World Health Organization, IPCS/Interregional Research Unit (IRRU), USA

PREFACE

The International Programme on Chemical Safety (IPCS) was initiated in 1980 as a collaborative programme of the United Nations Environment Programme (UNEP), the International Labour Organization (ILO) and the World Health Organization (WHO). One of the major objectives of the IPCS is to develop and evaluate principles and methodologies for assessing the effects of chemicals on human health and the environment. Since its inception, IPCS has been particularly concerned with assessing risk to the human reproductive system from exposure to chemicals and has given a high priority to improving methodologies and strategies in this area.

As part of this effort, IPCS publishes a series of monographs called Environmental Health Criteria (EHC). Past publications include two EHCs on aspects of risk assessment for reproductive health: EHC 30, "Principles for Evaluating Health Risks to Progeny Associated with Exposure to Chemicals during Pregnancy" (IPCS, 1984), and EHC 59, "Principles for Evaluating Health Risks from Chemicals during Infancy and Early Childhood: The Need for a Special Approach" (IPCS, 1986a). EHC 30 focused on the use of short-term tests and *in vivo* animal tests to assess prenatal toxicity and postnatal alterations in reproduction, development and behaviour following chemical exposure during gestation, and EHC 59 focused on methods to detect impaired reproductive and neurobehavioural development in infants and children who were exposed during the prenatal and early postnatal periods.

Many data and numerous new methods have emerged since these monographs were published in the 1980s, and the ability to assess the risk to reproductive health from chemical exposure has significantly improved. A number of urgent requests have been made by agencies in many different countries, particularly developing countries, for up-to-date information on principles and approaches to assessing reproductive health risk. In response to these requests, IPCS has produced another monograph on these issues. The present monograph focuses on approaches to assessing reproductive toxicity in males and females, including sexual dysfunction and infertility, and many aspects of developmental toxicity (following both prenatal and postnatal exposure), from conception to sexual maturation. It is an overview of the major scientific principles underlying hazard identification, testing methods and risk assessment strategies in human reproductive toxicity. It also discusses the evaluation of reproductive toxicity data in the context of the extensive risk assessment methodology that has emerged over the past 10–15 years.

IPCS is producing this monograph as a tool for use by public health officials, research and regulatory scientists and risk managers. It is intended to complement the monographs, reviews and test guidelines on reproductive and developmental toxicity currently available. However, this document does not provide specific guidelines or protocols for the application of risk assessment strategies or the conduct of specific tests. Specific testing guidelines for assessing reproductive toxicity from exposure to chemicals have been developed by the Organisation for Economic Co-operation and Development (OECD) and national governments.

Several meetings took place to discuss and evaluate the structure and content of this document. Initial drafts of the document were prepared by a group of authors (listed on the title page) and coordinated by the IPCS Secretariat, Dr B.-H. Chen and Dr T. Damstra. IPCS is grateful to these authors and acknowledges the time and expertise that they so generously gave to this project.

A preliminary draft was circulated for review to 52 experts in reproductive toxicology and IPCS contact points. Many reviewers provided substantive comments and text, and their contributions are gratefully acknowledged.

A Task Group meeting was held in Carshalton, United Kingdom, on 16–18 October 2000, to review a revised draft. Dr T. Damstra, IPCS, was responsible for the preparation of the final document and for its overall scientific content.

The efforts of all who helped in the preparation and finalization of the monograph are gratefully acknowledged. Special thanks are due to the US Environmental Protection Agency (EPA) and the Federal Ministry for the Environment, Nature Conservation and Nuclear Safety, Germany, for their financial support for the planning and review group meetings.

ACRONYMS AND ABBREVIATIONS

ABP	androgen binding protein
ACTH	adrenocorticotrophin hormone
ADI	allowable daily intake
ATPase	adenosine triphosphatase
AUC	area under the curve
bFGF	basic fibroblast growth factor
BMC	benchmark concentration
BMD	benchmark dose
BMP	bone morphogenetic protein
cAMP	cyclic adenosine monophosphate
C_{max}	maximum plasma concentration
CNS	central nervous system
DDE	dichlorodiphenyldichloroethylene
DDT	dichlorodiphenyltrichloroethane
DES	diethylstilbestrol
DHEA	dehydroepiandrosterone
DHEAS	dehydroepiandrosterone sulfate
DHT	dihydrotestosterone
DNA	deoxyribonucleic acid
DSP	daily sperm production
EC	European Commission
ECETOC	European Centre for Ecotoxicology and Toxicology of Chemicals
EDC	endocrine disrupting chemical
EGF	epidermal growth factor
Egr	early growth response
EHC	Environmental Health Criteria
EPA	Environmental Protection Agency (USA)
FAO	Food and Agriculture Organization of the United Nations
FDA	Food and Drug Administration (USA)
FGF	fibroblast growth factor
FSH	follicle stimulating hormone
GDF	growth differentiation factor
GnRH	gonadotrophin releasing hormone
HCB	hexachlorobenzene
hCG	human chorionic gonadotrophin
H-P-G axis	hypothalamic–pituitary–gonadal axis

hPL	human placental lactogen
HSD	hydroxysteroid dehydrogenase
IARC	International Agency for Research on Cancer
IC_{50}	median inhibitory concentration
ICM	inner cell mass
IGF	insulin-like growth factor
ILO	International Labour Organization
ILSI	International Life Sciences Institute
IPCS	International Programme on Chemical Safety
JECFA	Joint FAO/WHO Expert Committee on Food Additives
JMPR	Joint FAO/WHO Meeting on Pesticide Residues
K_i	inhibition rate constant
LDL	low-density lipoprotein
LH	luteinizing hormone
LOAEL	lowest-observed-adverse-effect level
MIS	Müllerian inhibiting substance
MOE	margin of exposure
NGF	nerve growth factor
NOAEL	no-observed-adverse-effect level
NTP	National Toxicology Program (USA)
OECD	Organisation for Economic Co-operation and Development
PAH	polycyclic aromatic hydrocarbon
PBB	polybrominated biphenyl
PCB	polychlorinated biphenyl
pK_a	negative log of the acid dissociation constant
QSAR	quantitative structure–activity relationship
RfC	reference concentration
RfD	reference dose
RNA	ribonucleic acid
SBR	standardized birth ratio
TDI	tolerable daily intake
TGF-alpha	transforming growth factor alpha
TGF-beta	transforming growth factor beta
UN	United Nations
UNEP	United Nations Environment Programme
VEGF	vascular endothelial growth factor
WHO	World Health Organization

1. SUMMARY AND RECOMMENDATIONS

1.1 Summary

Since the publication of the IPCS Environmental Health Criteria documents dealing with aspects of reproductive toxicity risk assessment in the early 1980s, new scientific data and methodologies have significantly improved the ability to assess how environmental chemicals may adversely affect the reproductive system. This progress is reflected in the availability of a number of national and international (e.g., Organisation for Economic Co-operation and Development) reproductive and developmental toxicity test guidelines, risk assessment guidelines and guidance documents, as well as some international test method validation studies. However, the potential for human exposure to environmental contaminants (via a variety of routes) to affect the function of the reproductive system and normal development remains an area of global concern.

Normal human reproduction is regulated by a finely tuned system of coordinated signals that direct the activity of multiple interdependent target cells, leading to the formation of gametes, their transport, release, fertilization, implantation and gestation, and, ultimately, the development of offspring that is eventually capable of successfully repeating the entire process under similar or different environmental conditions.

Throughout the entire life cycle, all aspects of reproductive function are dependent on various endocrine communicating systems that employ a wide variety of protein/peptide and steroid hormones, growth factors and other signalling molecules that affect target cell gene expression and/or protein synthesis. In particular, development and gametogenesis are regulated by a myriad of signals delivered in appropriate strength at precisely defined times. Although recent animal studies demonstrate that the developing fetus may be more sensitive to the effects of exposure to environmental chemicals than the adult system, effects may not be manifest until adulthood. Further characterization of the molecular mechanisms regulating the various aspects of normal reproduction and development is critical to our understanding of the variety of mechanisms through which exogenous chemicals may disrupt normal reproduction and development.

Sexual function and fertility reflect a wide variety of functions that are necessary for reproduction and may be affected by exposure to environmental factors. Any disturbance in the integrity of the reproductive system may affect these functions. Patterns of reported infertility vary around the world, but approximately 10% of all couples experience infertility at some time during their reproductive years. Human studies on altered sexual function/fertility provide the most direct means of assessing risk, but data are often unavailable. For many environmental chemicals, it is still necessary to rely on information derived from experimental animal models and laboratory studies.

In vivo animal studies for reproductive toxicity risk assessment typically utilize standard laboratory rodents. Fertility assessments in male animals have limited sensitivity as measures of reproductive injury, because, unlike humans, males of most test species produce sperm in numbers that greatly exceed the minimum requirements for fertility. Histopathological data on reproductive tissues play an important role in male reproductive toxicity risk assessment. Chemicals with estrogenic or antiandrogenic activity have been identified that are capable of causing reproductive effects in males. While sensitivity may differ, it is likely that mechanisms of action for these endocrine disrupting agents will be consistent or similar across mammalian species. For females, all functions of the reproductive system are under endocrine control and can be susceptible to disruption by effects on the reproductive endocrine system. However, single measurements of hormonal changes may be insensitive indicators of any damage because of large normal variability in females.

A variety of *in vitro* test systems, including isolated perfused testis/ovary, primary cultures of gonadal cells, investigation of subcellular fractions of different organs and cell types and *in vitro* fertilization techniques, are available that can be used in supplementary investigational studies of different aspects of the reproductive system. *In vitro* testing systems are especially useful for screening for toxicity potential and for identifying potential mechanisms of action of potential toxicants. However, these tests are limited in their ability to assess complex, integrative reproductive functions.

2

Developmental toxicity, defined in its widest sense to include any adverse effect on normal development either before or after birth, has become of increasing concern in recent years. Developmental toxicity can result from exposure of either parent prior to conception, from exposure of the embryo or fetus *in utero* or from exposure of the progeny after birth. Adverse developmental effects may be detected at any point in the life span of the organism. In addition to structural abnormalities, examples of manifestations of developmental toxicity include fetal loss, altered growth, functional defects, latent onset of adult disease, early reproductive senescence and shortened life span.

In vivo studies on pregnant experimental animals and their progeny have been widely used in developmental toxicity assessment. The aim of the maternal observations is to assess the relative contribution of maternal toxicity to any observed embryo/fetal toxicity. Observations on progeny include early and late embryonic deaths (resorptions), fetal weight, external malformations, visceral and skeletal anomalies and sex determination. Background information and historical records on abnormal development of the experimental animals are important for adequate interpretation of such toxicity studies. Functions that can be evaluated postnatally include neurological development, simple and complex behaviours, reproduction, endocrine function, immune competence, xenobiotic metabolism and physiological function of different organ systems. Latent manifestations of toxicity may include transplacental carcinogenicity (neoplasia in the progeny resulting from maternal exposure to chemical agents during pregnancy) and shortened life span. A wide range of *in vitro* systems, ranging from whole embryo culture through organ and tissue culture to a variety of non-mammalian systems, has also been developed for the study of developmental toxicity. *In vitro* tests are useful in investigation of mechanisms of normal and abnormal development to obtain information on dose–response relationships and specific organ toxicity, and perhaps as screening systems for selection or prioritization of chemicals for further *in vivo* studies.

The most feasible end-points for evaluating developmental toxicity in humans are vital status at birth (including embryo/fetal loss), readily identifiable congenital anomalies, gestational length, birth weight and sex ratio. Measurable postnatal developmental effects include changes in growth, behaviour and organ or system function, as well as cancer. Both prenatal and postnatal effects may not be apparent

3

until well after birth, and some may not appear until adulthood. For example, some congenital anomalies are not immediately apparent, and the long-term sequelae of intrauterine growth retardation are just now being appreciated. Chemical exposure during development may also affect the later reproductive function of the offspring. For example, chemicals could damage female germ cells *in utero* and affect the mature female's fertility; similarly, male stem cells or Sertoli cells could be depleted, potentially affecting sperm production.

Many countries have developed risk assessment processes for reproductive and developmental toxicity in order to set standards and regulate exposures. These processes typically include components of hazard identification, dose–response relationships, exposure assessment and risk characterization. Experimental testing protocols are largely based on identifying structural anomalies and/or functional deficits following chemical exposure during critical windows of the reproductive cycle. All available sources of animal and human data should be considered to assess specific reproductive and developmental toxic effects. Approaches for evaluating and summarizing reproductive toxicity data have improved. Nevertheless, assumptions must often be made in the risk assessment process because of gaps in knowledge about underlying biological processes and species differences. Risk assessment test methods and strategies need to be continually refined as new data and technologies become available.

1.2 Recommendations

In order to employ effective control and intervention strategies to prevent reproductive and developmental toxicity, an adequate knowledge base must be developed. The following recommendations are made to improve this knowledge base:

1. Establish and develop better (molecular) markers of effects on reproduction and development. Those that may have a human and animal congruence would be particularly useful and would aid in the evaluation and use of animal data in human risk assessment.

2. Examine the utility of newer technologies related to gene expression (e.g., gene arrays, proteomics, laser capture microscopy) to aid in the understanding and elucidation of the underlying

mechanisms of normal and abnormal reproductive function and development.

3. Strengthen and refine methods to assess both the critical windows of exposure through the entire spectrum of development and stages of development most vulnerable to manifestations of adverse effects.

4. Increase basic knowledge of the mechanisms of male reproductive physiology to a level comparable to the current level of knowledge on mechanisms of female reproductive physiology.

5. Promote the application of cellular and molecular understanding of gonadal and gamete functions to extend the understanding of toxicological effects on these tissues.

6. Search for and validate animal models to analyse toxicological aspects of reproductive biology to develop appropriate systems that are reproducible, low cost and easier to extrapolate to human disease.

7. Improve and validate *in vitro* methods for assessing mechanisms of potential reproductive toxicity.

8. Develop more accurate and efficient methods of measuring human exposure to environmental chemicals with potential reproductive toxicity.

9. Improve the surveillance, collection and harmonization of data on the frequency and geographical distribution of birth defects and developmental disorders, with special attention to establishment of complete registries.

10. Promote research efforts to better identify subpopulations potentially vulnerable to the effects of agents responsible for reproductive toxicity and to characterize the factors contributing to increased vulnerability.

11. In view of the sensitivity of the developing organism, place more emphasis on toxicity studies involving gestational and perinatal exposure to a chemical or mixture of chemicals.

12. Utilize previously studied birth cohorts to investigate the incidence of latent adverse reproductive outcomes later in life (cohorts with pregnancy exposure data are extremely important).

13. Establish an international harmonized system for terminology and definitions for reproductive and developmental toxicity.

2. INTRODUCTION

A growing body of scientific evidence indicates that exposure to a wide range of environmental contaminants causes adverse reproductive effects in humans and other species. These issues are a prominent public health concern of scientists, decision-makers and the general public. Many disorders of reproduction have been described in both males and females. Examples include reduced fertility, menstrual disorders, impaired spermatogenesis, cryptorchidism and hypospadias, pregnancy loss, low birth weight, structural and functional birth defects, postnatal developmental defects and various genetic diseases affecting the reproductive system and offspring. It has been estimated that the incidence of easily recognized birth defects is 2–3% of live births and that the incidence of less easily recognized birth defects and developmental disorders is 5–10% of live births from all causes (ICH, 1993).

The magnitude of reproductive problems in the general population is becoming widely recognized, and the possible role of environmental agents in causing these disorders has renewed worldwide interest in reproductive and developmental toxicology. Recently, the US National Toxicology Program (NTP) established the Center to Evaluate Risks to Human Reproduction, the purpose of which is to conduct risk assessment on agents with potential to cause reproductive and developmental toxicity.

This monograph summarizes current scientific knowledge on hazard identification and risk assessment for reproductive toxicity. For the purposes of this document, reproductive toxicity includes adverse effects on sexual function and fertility in males and females as well as developmental toxicity. This monograph builds on previously published Environmental Health Criteria monographs (EHCs) and scientific reviews (e.g., IPCS, 1984, 1986a; Moore, 1995; Moore et al., 1995; ILSI, 1999; US NRC, 2000). The document is intended as a tool for use by public health officials, research and regulatory scientists and risk managers. It seeks to provide a scientific framework for the use and interpretation of reproductive toxicity data from human and animal studies. It also discusses emerging methodology and testing strategy in reproductive toxicity.

Chapter 3 discusses basic reproductive physiology and the relative vulnerability of specific reproductive structures and processes and provides the scientific background for understanding specific methods and procedures used in reproductive toxicology. Chapter 4 focuses on methods for assessing and evaluating altered sexual function and fertility. Chapter 5 addresses methodologies for assessing developmental toxicity, defined as any effect interfering with normal development both before and after birth resulting from exposure of either parent prior to conception, exposure during prenatal development or exposure postnatally to the time of sexual maturation. Chapter 6 deals with the general principles of risk assessment for reproductive toxicity and identifies areas where research is needed. An appendix provides working definitions for the terminology used in the monograph.

A particular area of concern in reproductive and development toxicity relates to the effects of chemicals that have the potential to disrupt or interfere with the endocrine system (i.e., potential endocrine disrupting chemicals, or EDCs). The potential adverse health consequences of exposure to EDCs have fuelled intense public debate and media attention, and a considerable amount of scientific research is being conducted on EDCs. The concern over EDCs extends to governments, international organizations, scientific societies, the chemical industry and public interest groups. Many research programmes, conferences, workshops and committees are trying to address EDC-related issues. Endocrine disruption is only one of a diverse number of mechanisms for potentially causing adverse reproductive and developmental effects.

It is beyond the scope of this document to review the large body of data dealing with EDCs, and the reader is referred to recent comprehensive reviews (Colborn et al., 1996; US EPA, 1997b; Crisp et al., 1998; IUPAC, 1998; Olsson et al., 1998; US NRC, 1999). Also, at the request of international bodies, IPCS is preparing a "Global Assessment of the State-of-the-Science of Endocrine Disruptors" (in preparation) and has developed a Global Endocrine Disruptor Research Inventory. The US Environmental Protection Agency (EPA), Organisation for Economic Co-operation and Development (OECD) and a number of countries and industrial associations are implementing activities and collaborating on the development and validation of screening and testing methods to assess chemicals for their ability to disrupt the endocrine system (ECETOC, 1996; Ankley et al., 1998; US EPA, 1998d; OECD, 1999a, 1999b). These tests are referred to only briefly in this document.

As described in the Preface, this monograph does not provide practical advice or specific guidance for the conduct of specific tests and studies. These have been developed and issued by international organizations and national governments and vary with the types of chemicals being assessed and according to national regulations and recommendations. For example, the OECD has developed internationally agreed upon test guidelines for the reproductive toxicity testing of pesticides and industrial chemicals. The OECD is an intergovernmental organization of 29 industrialized countries in North America, Europe and the Pacific, as well as the European Commission, which meet to coordinate and harmonize policies and work together to respond to international concerns, including the effects of chemicals on human health and the environment.

Test guidelines specifically developed for reproductive toxicity testing in laboratory animals include Test Guideline 414 on prenatal developmental toxicity (OECD, 2001a), which was originally published as a guideline for teratogenicity studies (OECD, 1981a); Test Guideline 415 on one-generation reproductive toxicity (OECD, 1983a); Test Guideline 416 on two-generation reproductive toxicity (OECD, 1983b, 2001b); Test Guideline 421 on reproduction/developmental toxicity screening (OECD, 1995); and Test Guideline 422 on the combined repeated-dose toxicity study with reproduction/developmental toxicity screening (OECD, 1996b). An OECD guidance document on reproductive toxicity testing is also in preparation. Extensive risk assessment guidelines for reproductive toxicity testing have also been published by the US EPA (1996b, 1998b, 1998c) and the European Commission (EC, 1996). For pharmaceuticals and food additives, international bodies and national governments have also developed testing protocols (US FDA, 1982, 1993; IPCS, 1987). The harmonized guidelines for the safety testing of drugs are discussed briefly in chapter 5, since drug regulations are more advanced in their scientific development and reflect basic underlying principles similar to those for testing other types of chemicals (ICH, 1993). The reader should refer to these test guidelines for details and guidance on specific test protocols.

The testing of chemicals for reproductive toxicity is a dynamic and evolving process. As the basic sciences of molecular biology, reproductive physiology and endocrinology advance, so do the requirements for safety and risk evaluation. It must be emphasized that the design and interpretation of reproductive tests and the conduct of risk assessment on reproductive toxicity from exposure to environmental chemicals are a highly specialized science. Therefore, it is essential that properly trained professional reproductive toxicologists and epidemiologists conduct and interpret the results of such studies. It is hoped that this monograph will be a useful tool in this process.

3. PHYSIOLOGY OF HUMAN REPRODUCTION

3.1   Introduction

Human reproduction is regulated by a set of hormone signals that act in a finely tuned and coordinated manner. These hormones act upon multiple interdependent target cells, directing the development of germ line gametes as well as their transport, release, fertilization, implantation and gestation. This process produces offspring and continues indefinitely, maintaining the evolutionary survival of the species. As indicated in chapter 2, exposures to certain environmental contaminants can adversely influence reproduction and development through a variety of mechanisms. Therefore, it is important to improve our understanding of the impact of such exposures on human reproductive health.

This chapter focuses on the endocrine organ communication system and its regulation of human reproduction and development and describes the major endocrine regulating elements and their anatomical and functional characteristics. Other molecular and cellular events and signalling pathways also play a major role, but are not discussed here. The critical developmental stages and the basic physiological processes of reproduction and fetal development are emphasized, with separate discussion of processes and elements important during adulthood and pre- and postnatal development. The principal elements important during adulthood (Figure 1) are gamete production and release, fertilization, zygote transport, growth and development, sexual maturation and reproductive senescence. During pre- and postnatal stages (Figure 1), the elements are implantation, embryogenesis, fetal development, parturition, lactation and postnatal development. The possible influences of environmental contaminants on human reproduction and development are discussed throughout the chapter.

3.2   Reproductive endocrinology

3.2.1   Gonadal function

A central concept and mechanism in reproductive and developmental biology is hormonal communication. Small-molecule hormones

The Reproductive Cycle

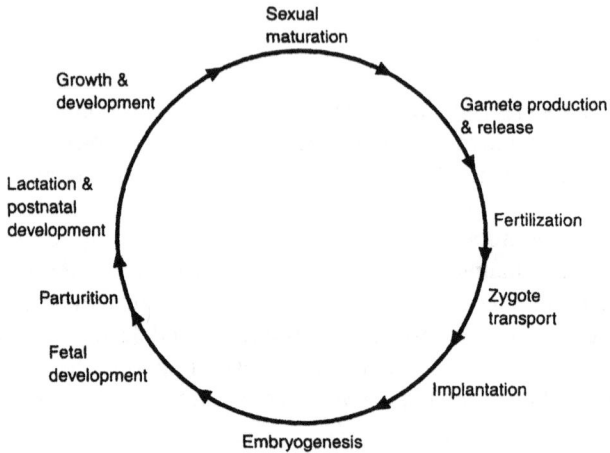

Fig. 1. Diagram of the major reproductive life cycle phases, commencing with sexual maturation and moving through fertilization, fetal development, parturition and postnatal development and ending with a sexually mature individual capable of starting the cycle over again.

communicate information from the endocrine glands to the cells of target tissues located throughout the body, thereby regulating fetal and postnatal development as well as production and release of gametes. It is essential for normal reproductive function and fetal development that appropriate hormone signals reach target tissues at the proper time. Hormones convey information to cells that are proximal or distal to the site of synthesis and secretion. When a hormone targets the cell from which it was secreted, it is termed autocrine hormone signalling; if the target is a different cell in the same tissue, it is termed paracrine hormone signalling. Peptide hormones recognize and activate membrane-bound receptors on the surface of the target cell; downstream events can involve one or more signalling cascades (i.e., activation of adenylate cyclase, higher cAMP level, increased enzyme activity). In contrast, steroid hormones are highly lipophilic and can cross cellular membranes into the cytoplasm or nucleus, where they recognize appropriate receptor molecules that can regulate transcription, translation or protein synthesis.

The integration and coordination of the effects of peptide and steroid hormones require delicate and precise control. Together, these two types of hormones provide the mechanisms by which the endocrine system regulates complex cellular pathways, such as cell division, differentiation, protein and steroid synthesis and programmed cell death, as well as reproduction and development. Many steps in hormone action can affect reproductive function and fetal development; these steps include hormone production, release, transport, metabolism, receptor binding, postreceptor events and intracellular events such as DNA binding. The complete cellular and molecular details of the mechanisms directing these events are beyond the scope of the discussion in this chapter; however, the interested reader is referred to reports and reviews referenced throughout the text.

The hypothalamus, pituitary and gonads (the hypothalamic–pituitary–gonadal, or H-P-G, axis) are the basic endocrine elements that regulate the reproductive system (Figure 2). Although anatomically discrete, these structures are functionally linked to each other. Regulation of the H-P-G axis and communication between its elements depend on hormone levels and sensitive feedback control mechanisms. Peptide and steroid hormones stimulate the gonads, which then produce steroid hormones that act locally on the gonad itself in an autocrine and paracrine manner. These hormones also function in a classical endocrine manner on accessory sex organs, such as the mammary gland and uterus in women and the epididymis and prostate in men. Gonadal hormones also effect negative feedback on the hypothalamus and pituitary and inhibit gene transcription, translation and synthesis of the decapeptide gonadotrophin releasing hormone (GnRH) and pituitary gonadotrophins luteinizing hormone (LH) and follicle stimulating hormone (FSH). In women, estradiol effects positive feedback on the hypothalamus and pituitary at ovulation, which elevates the circulating level of LH.

The gonads produce steroid hormones, including progestins, androgens and estrogens. These steroid hormones play a significant role in regulating reproductive processes, including sexual development, production and release of gametes, fertilization, pregnancy, fetal development, parturition, the development of secondary sexual characteristics and lactation. Most of the enzymes that synthesize gonadal steroids are members of the cytochrome P-450 superfamily of oxidases and are located in the smooth endoplasmic reticulum of steroidogenic

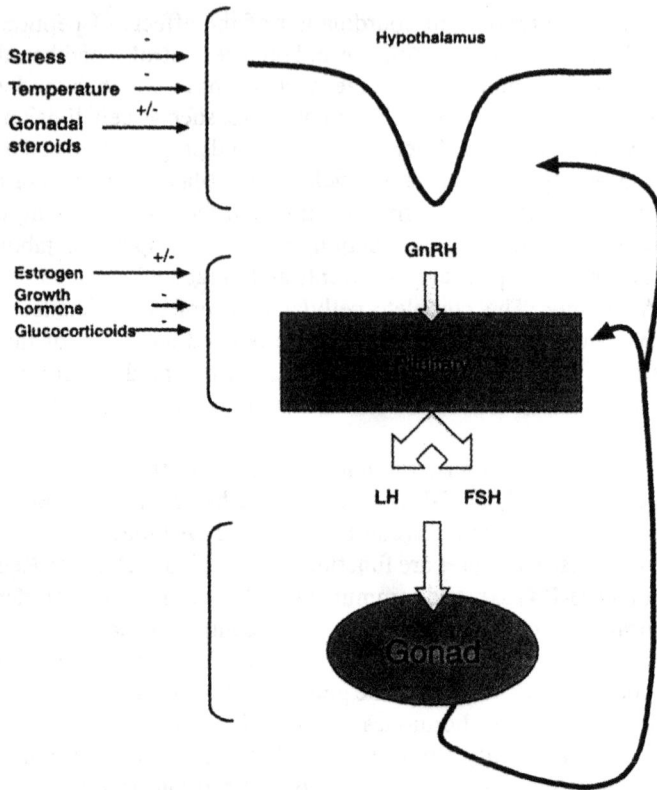

Fig. 2. Gonadotrophin releasing hormone (GnRH) released in pulses by the hypothalamus stimulates pituitary production and secretion of luteinizing hormone (LH) and follicle stimulating hormone (FSH). The hypothalamic–pituitary—gonadal (H-P-G) axis is affected by a variety of external hormones and external factors.

cells. However, conversion of cholesterol to pregnenolone by cytochrome P-450 side-chain cleavage occurs in mitochondria. Steroidogenesis follows two different pathways (Figure 3); the choice between the Δ^4 or the Δ^5 pathway depends on the availability of substrate and enzymes, as well as the tissue and the species. For example, unlike the gonads, the placenta is unable to convert cholesterol to progestins because it lacks the required enzymes. Also, the Δ^4 pathway dominates in the testis in the rat, whereas the Δ^5 pathway is the major route of testosterone synthesis in the rabbit. These differences must be considered when using animal models to predict effects in humans.

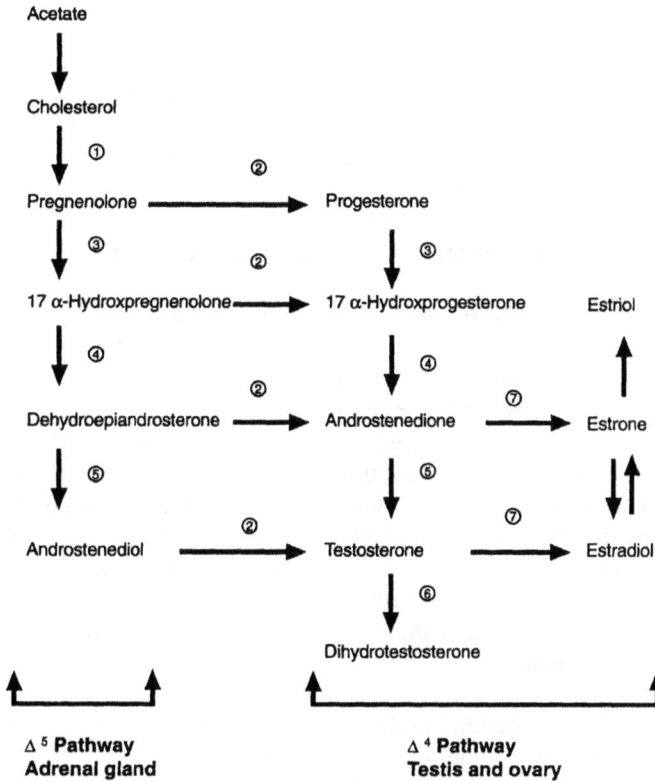

Fig. 3. Gonadal steroid biosynthetic pathway and the catalytic enzymes: 1) cytochrome P-450scc; 2) 3β-hydroxysteroid dehydrogenase; 3) 17α-hydroxylase (P-450scc17); 4) 17,20-desmolase or 17,20-lyase; 5) 17β-hydroxysteroid dehydrogenase; 6) 5α-reductase; and 7) P-450 aromatase.

The gonads also contain enzymes that carry out biotransformation and detoxification to protect the gonads from damage due to oxidative stress or exogenous chemicals. Cytochrome P-450 enzymes carry out phase I biotransformation reactions, producing water-soluble products that readily undergo phase II biotransformation reactions (Sipes & Gandolfi, 1991). Enzymes that protect the gonads from such damage (phase II detoxification enzymes) include glutathione peroxidase, glutathione reductase, superoxide dismutase and catalase. In animal experiments, these defence mechanisms can be overwhelmed by treatment with chemicals such as polychlorinated biphenyls (PCBs), 7,12-dimethylbenz[a]anthracene or hexachlorobenzene (HCB). In some cases, the effects of these chemicals include structural alteration of mitochondria of ovarian granulosa cells, uncoupling of oxidative phosphorylation and altered steroidogenesis. These experiments and other data suggest that environmental contaminants can reduce circulating steroid levels by decreasing the level of pituitary gonadotrophins (Müller et al., 1978; Foster, 1992; Jansen et al., 1993). In addition, direct effects on steroidogenic enzyme activity have been observed (Drew & Miners, 1984; Evenson & Jost, 1993).

3.2.2 Basic elements underlying normal development

Embryonic development is arguably the most complicated of biological processes. It involves the formation of a new individual from a single cell, the fertilized zygote. A high rate of cell division is the most obvious of the events that must take place in order for development to occur, but it is far from the only one. Formation of the embryo from the mass of cells accumulating from repeated cell division involves the establishment of three germ layers of body axes (anterior–posterior, ventral–dorsal, left–right), the partitioning of groups of cells into organ primordia and the development of those primordia into discrete structures.

A number of cellular and molecular mechanisms underlie these processes. These include intercellular communication, governed by paracrine and endocrine factors (hormones and growth factors); cell surface and extracellular matrix proteins that control migration and mutual induction between discrete groups of cells; selective expression and suppression of genes, leading to differentiation of cells; and a balance of cell proliferation and programmed cell death (apoptosis) to provide an ample number of cells for organ development and to establish form. While these events are going on, the embryo is also undergoing marked changes in intermediary metabolism, progressing from mostly glycolytic to mostly oxidative as the placenta and embryonic circulatory system become functional, and xenobiotic metabolism. All of these processes are essential for normal development, and any may be a target for exogenous insult that may lead to abnormal development.

The literature on these processes and their role in normal and abnormal development is too large to review here, but is important for understanding normal and abnormal development. The reader is directed to a recent compendium on mechanisms of abnormal development (Kavlock & Daston, 1997).

3.3 Female reproductive physiology

.3.1 *Ovarian development and oogenesis*

The principal functions of the ovary are to produce ova, gonadal steroids (estrogens and progestin) and other hormones, such as inhibin and activin. Numerous other factors, such as cytokines, prostaglandins and growth factors, are also produced by the ovary to regulate follicular development (folliculogenesis), ovulation or luteal function in an autocrine or paracrine fashion. Cyclical ovarian function also regulates the menstrual cycle in women and the estrous cycle in female rats. The endocrine regulation of ovarian function, menstrual cycle and follicular development has been reviewed previously (Erickson, 1978; Goebelsmann, 1986; Ferin, 1996).

Oogenesis is the process of ovum formation and maturation. During oogenesis, primordial germ cells are formed, which become oogonia and subsequently oocytes in the fetus. In the adult, oocytes mature into ova, which contain the nutrients that support the early embryo's energy requirements (Wasserman, 1996; Wasserman & Albertini, 1996).

In the female fetus, primordial germ cells are formed from stem cells in the yolk sac endoderm, and these cells are the sole source of germ cells in the adult. The primordial germ cells migrate to the genital ridges and subsequently into the cortex of the developing ovary, where, together with the superficial epithelium, they give rise to the cortical sex cords of the ovary. Once the developing ovary forms, the primordial germ cells are converted to oogonia, which divide mitotically until approximately 6–7 million oogonia are formed at approximately 20 weeks of gestation. At this time, the oogonia enter meiosis, and the number of oocytes is fixed (Baker, 1963). Oogonia are transformed into oocytes when the last mitotic division occurs in preparation for meiosis. Once oocytes enter the diplotene phase of meiosis, they become arrested, also called the dictyate stage, and remain in that stage until meiosis resumes at ovulation. The oocytes remain arrested in meiosis I until the preovulatory surge of LH (Baker, 1982).

From the 20th week of gestation until puberty, the ovary is composed primarily of primordial follicles, each of which possesses an oocyte arrested in the first meiotic cell division surrounded by a single flattened layer of granulosa cells. A number of these follicles begin to develop spontaneously, becoming a primary follicle; in the absence of gonadotrophin, however, they undergo apoptosis. The number of primordial follicles continues to decline due to apoptosis from the 20th week of gestation until reproductive senescence or menopause.

At the time of menarche or puberty, there may be only 300 000 – 400 000 oocytes in the ovaries. With the onset of puberty, a second layer begins to form from cuboidal granulosa cells; these cells arise from a small number of growing follicles that have an enlarged ooplasm and a zona pellucida.

3.3.2 *Functional morphology of the ovary*

The ovary is the source of the female gametes and the reproductive hormones that regulate the female reproductive cycle. The adult ovary is made up of the cortex (containing ovarian follicles), the medulla and the hilum (the ovarian attachment area). The medulla consists of the ovarian stroma, which are mainly connective tissue, and the sex steroid-producing interstitial cells. A follicle progresses from an inactive primordial follicle to a preovulatory Graafian follicle in approximately 2 months. Only the last 2–3 weeks of this maturation process is responsive to and controlled by the pituitary gonadotrophins LH and FSH. Throughout the female reproductive life, maturing follicles undergo atresia at different stages.

Structurally, the ovary is composed of germinal epithelium, ovarian follicles in different stages of development and stromal tissue. The functional unit of the ovary is the follicle, which is a single oocyte surrounded by granulosa cells, a basement membrane and a thin layer of thecal cells. During folliculogenesis, granulosa cells proliferate, an antrum develops containing granulosa cell secretions and the follicle enlarges. Following ovulation, the corpus luteum forms, which either persists during pregnancy or regresses to form a corpus albicans in the absence of fertilization.

1.2.1   Folliculogenesis

As mentioned above, oocytes are arrested in the diplotene phase of the first meiotic division before sexual maturity is reached. Follicles begin maturing in the presence of low circulating levels of estradiol (Erickson, 1978; Goebelsmann, 1986), but gonadotrophin is not required. As a population of follicles begins to grow, a single follicle is selected to become the dominant follicle for ovulation. The oocyte enlarges and the granulosa cells become cuboidal and thicken to three or more layers. This is now called a secondary follicle.

While the oocyte remains constant in size, the granulosa cells undergo rapid division, and a fluid-filled antrum forms. Such a Graafian or antral follicle is 5–6 times larger than the secondary follicle. The innermost layer of granulosa cells surrounding the oocyte (the corona radiata) becomes columnar, and these cells form specialized gap junctions with the oocyte plasma membrane that are important in regulation of oocyte development. The oocyte secretes a layer of glycoproteins to form the zona pellucida, which separates the oocyte from the surrounding corona radiata. The layer of cells and connective tissue that envelops and delineates the follicle from the surrounding ovarian stroma is the theca. The dominant follicle grows at a faster rate and produces a higher level of estradiol than the remainder of the growing pool of follicles. Serum FSH induces expression of LH receptors on the surface of thecal cells, which then produce pregnenolone, progesterone and, subsequently, androstenedione. Androstenedione is transported into granulosa cells, where it is converted first to testosterone by 17-hydroxysteroid dehydrogenase and then to estradiol via an irreversible reaction catalysed by the enzyme P-450 aromatase (Figure 4). While the remaining developing follicles become apoptotic, the granulosa cells of the dominant follicle continue to divide, eventually producing an antrum within the follicle.

The rising level of estradiol that results from folliculogenesis leads to a mid-cycle surge in LH, which induces the dominant follicle to ovulate. In preparation for fertilization, meiosis is resumed, forming one daughter cell and one small polar body. The daughter cell enters the second meiotic division and arrests in the second metaphase until fertilization. The follicle becomes highly vascularized, the follicular wall forms a protrusion (macula pellucida) where rupture occurs and the oocyte and its surrounding granulosa cells are released. At

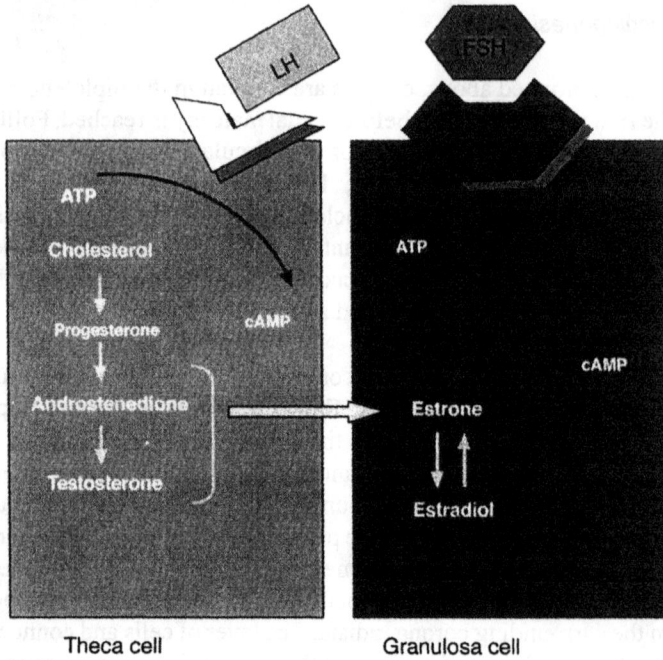

Fig. 4. The gonadotrophin two-cell model of ovarian steroidogenesis involves the stimulation of thecal cells by LH to produce androstenedione and testosterone while FSH stimulates granulosa cells to synthesize estrogens from the theca-derived androgens.

ovulation, the oocyte is extruded onto the ovarian surface, where the cumulus mass can be retrieved by the fimbriated end of the fallopian tube. Once the oocyte has been extruded at ovulation, the nucleus progresses from the dictyate stage of the first meiotic division (2N) to metaphase II (1N), where it remains until fertilized.

After ovulation, the walls of the follicular cavity in the ovary develop into the corpus luteum, which persists if fertilization occurs or disintegrates if fertilization does not occur. In addition to triggering ovulation, the mid-cycle surge in LH induces luteinization of the thecal and granulosa cells of the follicle wall. Normal luteal function depends upon both normal folliculogenesis and successful follicular rupture. Vascularization of the follicle wall with ovulation makes it possible for the luteinized thecal and granulosa cells to access low-density lipoprotein (LDL) cholesterol circulating in the blood; cholesterol is required for synthesis of progesterone.

Inhibin is produced by granulosa cells and exerts negative feed-back on the serum FSH level in the female. Inhibin is composed of a single *a* chain and two distinct *b* chains designated as bA and bB. Dimers containing bA or bB are called inhibin A and inhibin B, respectively. During the first half of the menstrual cycle, inhibin B is the dominant form in the serum; during the second half of the cycle, inhibin A is the dominant form. Thus, the appearance of inhibin A correlates well with the decline in the circulating level of FSH in the luteal phase of the cycle. The hormone activin is also produced by granulosa cells in the female and stimulates FSH, although autocrine action of the pituitary-derived activin may be more important. Activins are composed of two different subunits that form homodimers AA and BB or a heterodimer AB. These three forms are called activin A, activin B and activin AB, respectively. Like the inhibins, activins are widely produced in different tissues.

Throughout postpubertal life, cohorts of follicles are recruited. Some of these mature to become Graafian follicles and ovulate; however, most follicles undergo atresia. Although approximately 1 million follicles are present in the ovaries at birth, essentially all are depleted by about the age of 50 years, resulting in menopause. Toxicants can have many adverse effects on ovarian function, including a decrease in the number of primordial follicles, death of follicles, disrupted steroid-ogenesis or delayed ovulation (see chapter 4). The mechanisms of action of ovarian toxicants are not well defined but may include hor-mone mimicry or increase in oxygen free radicals and uncoupling of oxidative phosphorylation (Foster et al., 1995).

3.3.2.2   *Intraovarian signalling*

The principal extraovarian regulators of intraovarian processes are the pituitary gonadotrophins LH and FSH. Within the ovary, andro-gens, estrogens and progestins are important *in situ* regulators. Receptors for all three gonadal steroids are present in the ovary, suggesting that intraovarian signalling occurs via classical steroid hormone–receptor mechanisms. Androgens exert actions on the granu-losa cells, are used to produce estrogen, induce aromatase activity and promote progestin synthesis (Armstrong & Dorrington, 1976; Lucky et al., 1977).

Androgens also promote follicular atresia in the absence of gonadotrophins and generally oppose estrogen action. The thecal cells and the interstitial cells of the ovarian stroma produce androgens under the influence of LH. Circulating LDL cholesterol is converted to pregnenolone, then to progesterone. The 17α-hydroxylase/17,20-desmolase activity in the thecal/interstitial cells is responsible for converting pregnenolone and progesterone to dehydroepiandrosterone (DHEA) and androstenedione. The androgen produced is mainly androstenedione, which can go directly into the circulation, be converted to testosterone or be aromatized to estrogens in the granulosa cells by FSH-induced aromatase activity. This compartmentalized production of steroids (androgen substrate in thecal cells, estrogens in granulosa cells) should be kept in mind when considering results from *in vitro* cultures of granulosa or thecal cells. These cells have distinct gonadotrophin receptors (LH receptors in thecal cells; FSH receptors in granulosa cells) and enzyme activities, all of which are needed for estrogen production. *In vivo*, these cells function cooperatively.

Estrogens promote cellular division in the granulosa cells, prevent follicular atresia, enhance antrum formation and inhibit ovarian androgen production. Because regulation of all ovarian processes cannot be explained adequately by gonadal steroids alone, it is likely that other intraovarian regulators exist. Such putative intraovarian regulators have to meet the following criteria: 1) be produced in the ovary; 2) have a receptor in the ovary; and 3) have a biological effect on the ovary. By these criteria, insulin-like growth factor-1 (IGF-1) is an intraovarian regulator. The ovary produces IGF-1, its receptor is found in the ovary and IGF-1 influences steroidogenesis in both granulosa and thecal cells (Adashi et al., 1989; Guthrie et al., 1995).

Other putative intraovarian regulators are epidermal growth factor (EGF) and transforming growth factor-alpha (TGF-alpha), which share the same receptor and may have autocrine and paracrine activities in the ovary. One of the primary actions of FSH is to increase the expression of LH/human chorionic gonadotrophin (hCG) receptors, and this effect is inhibited by EGF (May & Schomberg, 1989). EGF also has mitogenic effects on granulosa cells and may be an important signal for granulosa cell proliferation. TGF-alpha is thought to act similarly to EGF. Another putative intraovarian regulator is transforming growth factor-beta 1 (TFG-beta 1), which increases steroidogenesis in granulosa cells (Knecht et al., 1989) and decreases steroidogenesis in thecal (Knecht et al., 1989) and Leydig cells (Lin et al., 1987).

Acidic and basic fibroblast growth factor (bFGF) are related and act through the same receptor. bFGF may act during early embryogenesis to promote differentiation of ectoderm to mesoderm. bFGF may also promote development of follicles in preparation for ovulation before gonadotrophin dependence develops (Gospodarowicz, 1989). It also may mediate angiogenesis in follicular development (Koos, 1989).

Other possible ovarian regulators include tumour necrosis factor-alpha, catecholaminergic input, luteinization inhibitor, gonadotrophin-binding inhibitors, oocyte maturation inhibitor and the ovarian renin–angiotensin system. Ovarian renin–angiotensin has been detected in follicular fluid (Lightman et al., 1989).

Receptor sites for angiotensin II, the main active peptide of the renin–angiotensin system, have been found in the ovaries (Lightman et al., 1989). Ovarian renin–angiotensin may also have an autocrine role in angiogenesis, steroidogenesis and oocyte maturation. Inhibin is produced by the ovarian follicle and corpus luteum (Tsonis et al., 1987) and appears to have some autocrine action on thecal and granulosa cells involving steroidogenesis (Burger & Findlay, 1989). Evidence is growing that multiple other substances — i.e., vascular endothelial growth factor (VEGF) and growth differentiation factors (GDF) 9 and 9B — also influence intraovarian functions.

Two other putative intraovarian regulators are Müllerian inhibiting substance (MIS) and oocyte maturation inhibitor. MIS is produced by the Sertoli cells of the fetal testis; its function is to regress the Müllerian duct in the male fetus. Thus, it is the first hormonal determinant of male gonadal differentiation. Granulosa cells also produce MIS; however, by the time the primordial germ cells are primary follicles in the female fetus, the Müllerian duct becomes resistant to MIS. Although not well characterized, oocyte maturation inhibitor may arrest oocytes in the dictyate stage in the first meiotic division and in metaphase in the second meiotic division (Tsafriri & Adashi, 1994).

3.3.3 Neuroendocrine regulation of ovarian function and reproductive cycling

3.3.3.1 Hypothalamus

Beginning in fetal life, the release of GnRH from the hypo-thalamus stimulates production of LH and FSH by the pituitary. The mean peak plasma levels of LH and FSH during gestation are higher in the female than in the male fetus. The pulsatile release of LH and FSH is controlled by neurons in the arcuate nucleus of the hypothalamus, which secrete GnRH into the hypothalamic–hypophyseal portal system. Dopamine and serotonin are among the hypothalamic neurotransmitters important in this process. Estradiol provides both positive and negative feedback to control GnRH release.

The peptidergic neurons in the hypothalamus produce GnRH, which is released in a pulsatile fashion (Knobil, 1980) into the hypo-thalamic–hypophyseal portal circulation and transported to the anterior pituitary, where it binds to high-affinity receptors on the surface of pituitary gonadotrophs. Change in the pulse frequency of GnRH is the mechanism by which GnRH regulates the synthesis and secretion of both LH and FSH. Both LH and FSH are secreted in a pulsatile fashion in response to GnRH and are released into the cavernous sinuses that surround the pituitary and drain into the general circulation for trans-port to the gonads.

GnRH-containing neurons receive a variety of neural inputs that regulate GnRH release. Opioids, dopamine and serotonin decrease the pulse frequency of GnRH; in contrast, norepinephrine and, to a lesser extent, epinephrine increase GnRH pulse frequency. Disruption of the pulse generator system by factors that result in continuous GnRH release or repress secretion decrease pituitary gonadotrophin secretion and thus suppress gonadal function.

3.3.3.2 Pituitary

The pituitary gland is composed of anterior and posterior lobes that are attached to the hypothalamus via the infundibulum or hypo-physeal stalk, which includes the portal vessels. Processes from GnRH cells in the hypothalamus terminate on or in the vicinity of the portal vessels that convey blood to the anterior lobe of the pituitary. The anterior lobe of the pituitary is highly vascular and contains sinusoids, which are irregularly anastamosing terminal blood vessels consisting of a single layer of endothelial cells and a basement membrane. Primarily acidophilic, chromophobic and basophilic cells line the sinusoids. It is the latter cell type, the gonadotrophs, that are responsible for producing LH and FSH in response to stimulation by GnRH. These glycoprotein hormones are composed of two polypeptide chains designated α and β. The α chain is common to both LH and FSH, whereas the β chain differs and confers immunological and hormonal specificity. Experiments carried out with animal model systems indicate that environmental contaminants can alter pituitary function and the level of GnRH. For example, perfusion of pituitary glands *in vitro* with PCBs can influence synthesis and secretion of gonadotrophins (Jansen et al., 1993).

3.3.3   Patterns of ovarian response

The balanced secretion of FSH and LH controls follicular growth, ovulation and maintenance of pregnancy. Both hormones interact with cell surface receptors on their target cells in the ovary. In addition, FSH stimulates aromatization of theca-derived androgens to estrogens by granulosa cells (Gore-Langton & Armstrong, 1994). The main endocrine action of FSH is to stimulate granulosa cells to produce progesterone. LH stimulation induces follicular thecal cells and stromal interstitial cells to produce androgens. LH is secreted at a basal level in prepubertal females with irregular pulsatile occurrences. In human cycling females, the ovarian hormonal profile is linked to the menstrual cycle, which is controlled by LH and FSH levels. There is an LH surge before ovulation that is temporally linked to the preceding rise of estradiol. After ovulation, the levels of progesterone and, to a lesser extent, estrogen accelerate until luteolysis, when progesterone and estrogen levels return to basal values (Greenwald, 1987).

3.3.4   Effects of hormones on reproductive tract and breast

During pregnancy, progesterone, estrogen and prolactin stimulate proliferation of alveolar cells. Pulsatile secretion of gonadotrophins starts at puberty, and the subsequent increase in estrogen level stimulates growth of the rudimentary mammary gland. When progesterone is produced as part of an ovulatory cycle, it stimulates the alveolar buds within the mammary lobules. After puberty, the changing estrogen and progesterone levels in the cycling female affect breast tissue development, with maximal activity in the luteal phase. Since the levels of estrogen and progesterone in the cycling female are under the influence of the hypothalamo–pituitary axis, the neuroendocrine system indirectly influences breast development.

The signal for the breast to start producing milk after delivery is probably the rapid decline in serum concentration of progesterone and estrogen that occurs after delivery. Growth hormone, adrenocorticotrophin hormone (ACTH) and thyroxine are involved in maintaining lactation, and the hypothalamus regulates their production by the pituitary and thyroid gland, respectively.

3.4 Male reproductive physiology

3.4.1 Testes

The principal roles of the male gonads are to produce gonadal steroids and spermatozoa to fertilize the ovum. The gonadal steroid testosterone acts in a paracrine manner to stimulate spermatogenesis in the testis. From the early teen years until puberty in the male, the circulating level of gonadotrophin increases at night and induces the production of testosterone. In target tissues, testosterone is converted to dihydrotestosterone (DHT), which is a more potent androgen than testosterone and stimulates development of secondary sexual characteristics. Male accessory sex organs such as the prostate are incapable of synthesizing testosterone themselves.

The testes are composed of the interstitium and the seminiferous tubule, which are histologically distinct compartments. The interstitium is composed of nests of Leydig cells, which surround the seminiferous tubule and produce testosterone. The seminiferous tubule is the site of spermatogenesis and constitutes approximately 90% of the testis volume. The seminiferous tubule contains male germ cells in different stages of development and Sertoli (nurse) cells. Columnar Sertoli cells extend from the basement membrane to the lumen of the tubule. These cells form tight junctions in the basal region of the cells and thus form the anatomical basis for the blood–testis barrier, which divides the tubule into basal and adluminal compartments. Spermatogonia are located in the basal compartment, and the developing spermatocytes and maturing spermatids are located in the adluminal compartment.

The blood–testis barrier is an important structural element of the testis because it prevents large molecules, ions and steroid hormones from passing from the basal region into the adluminal compartment. The Sertoli cells are key structural elements in the seminiferous tubule and play a central role in spermatogenesis; they provide nutrients to the developing germ cells, translocate them to the lumen of the tubule and eliminate degenerating germ cells and their products.

FSH plays a key role in spermatogenesis; it binds G-protein-coupled membrane-bound receptors on Sertoli cells and induces the Sertoli cells to proliferate during pre- and postnatal development. FSH also induces Sertoli cells to produce androgen binding protein (ABP), TGF-beta 1, MIS and other important signalling compounds. Sertoli cells also play an important role in spermiation and are the source of the seminiferous tubule fluid that provides nutrients to sperm cells as they travel from the testis to the epididymis.

3.4.2 Spermatogenesis

Spermatogenesis is the process by which precursor cells form mature haploid spermatozoa within the seminiferous tubule. Spermatogonia multiply mitotically, but remain quiescent during most of the prepubertal period. After puberty, approximately 3 million spermatogonia begin to develop into spermatozoa each day (Johnson et al., 1983), and daily sperm production (DSP) is approximately 100 million. Spermatogenesis, which takes approximately 70 days and comprises the phases of spermatogonial proliferation, meiotic divisions of the spermatocytes and differentiation of spermatids (spermiogenesis) and spermatogenesis, has been reviewed previously (Sharpe, 1994; Matsumoto, 1996). During the proliferative phase of spermatogenesis, the spermatogonia that lie above the basement membrane but beneath the tight junctions at the basal region of Sertoli cells undergo a series of mitotic divisions. This renews the stem cell population and creates a group of germ cells that are committed to further cell division and differentiation.

In humans, there are only two type A spermatogonia (dark and pale) and one generation of type B spermatogonia; in rodents, there are several generations of type A spermatogonia plus intermediate and type B spermatogonia. Spermatogonia divide mitotically. After division of type B spermatogonia, preleptotent spermatocytes emerge. These cells undergo DNA replication and the first prophase of meiosis, which take more than 3 weeks in humans. After the first meiotic division, the second division rapidly follows without another S-phase, generating haploid germ cells called spermatids. Round spermatids undergo a complex morphogenetic process (spermiogenesis), including nuclear elongation and condensation, acrosome formation and flagellar development. This process ends up with release of mature spermatids to seminiferous tubular lumen (spermiation). After spermiation, the germ cells, which are now called spermatozoa, pass into the rete testis and further to the seminal pathway (Bustos-Obregõn et al., 1975).

During spermiogenesis, the third and last phase of spermatogenesis, spermatids become mature spermatozoa. The spermatids lose all excess cytoplasm, the nucleus loses fluid, the tail forms, the acrosome develops and the chromosomes condense. The nucleus moves to an eccentric position, and an acrosomal cap separates it from the cranial pole of the spermatozoa. The acrosome is closely attached to the spermatic cell membrane. The flagellum forms from centrioles at the caudal pole of the nucleus. The flagellum is divided into a middle, principal and end section. Mitochondria aggregate and form a spiral sheath around the middle of the flagellum. After the flagellum develops, the cytoplasm and its organelles reorganize, and the nucleus becomes condensed. Spermatids appear at the luminal surface of the seminiferous tubule and are released by a process called spermiation. The spermatozoa, which are still immature, are transported via the rete testis to the epididymis. On passage through the epididymis, the spermatozoa continue to mature. The mature spermatozoan is motile and can undergo the acrosome reaction.

Factors that alter the level of testosterone, by decreasing synthesis, increasing metabolic clearance or blocking the androgen receptor, can adversely affect the amount or quality of semen. It has been reported that exposure to environmental chemicals may lead to reduced semen quality (see chapter 4).

As discussed above, Sertoli cells play a central role in spermatogenesis. These cells also produce the regulatory molecules inhibin and activin, which are members of the TGF superfamily (see review by Vale et al., 1994). In males, activin and inhibin B coordinately regulate the level of serum FSH. Inhibin is a peptide hormone produced in response to FSH that exerts negative feedback on the pituitary gland to reduce serum FSH. Inhibin B is produced to a small extent in other tissues, but the level of inhibin B and the inhibin/FSH ratio can be useful indicators of Sertoli cell function. Activins are similar to inhibin, but they stimulate release of FSH from the pituitary. However, activin produced locally in the pituitary gland is more important in stimulating FSH secretion than activin secreted by the testes.

3.4.3   *Intratesticular signalling*

The main autocrine hormones in the testes are androgens, the most important of which is testosterone. As mentioned above, testosterone is converted to the more potent DHT in peripheral tissues. Testicular androgens produced by Leydig cells act locally to control spermatogenesis. Leydig cells store cholesterol in lipid droplets in their cytoplasm and use the cholesterol to form androgens.

Estrogens are also produced by Leydig cells and are able to inhibit spermatogenesis. In adult male rats, administration of estrogens suppresses spermatogenesis (Handelsman et al., 2000). This may result from estrogen-mediated suppression of LH, which decreases secretion of testosterone by Leydig cells, or it may indicate an intratesticular role for estradiol. It is likely that many of the factors involved in intraovarian signalling are involved in intratesticular signalling; for example, IGF-1 may regulate spermatogenesis (Antich et al., 1995). In the young rat, Sertoli cells can also convert androgens to estrogens (Sharpe et al., 1995).

Since FSH and LH are involved in spermatogenesis, hypothalamic control of their release by the pituitary is important for testicular function. Both FSH and LH are secreted in a pulsatile fashion from the pituitary. Inhibin B produced by Sertoli cells has the most important negative feedback effect on FSH secretion, while testosterone exerts negative feedback effects on secretion of GnRH by the hypothalamus, thus regulating secretion of LH and, to a lesser extent, FSH.

3.5   Mating behaviour

In human males and females, androgen increases libido. Women treated with androgens frequently experience increased libido, whereas women treated with antiandrogens experience reduced libido. Sexual activity may occur when testosterone levels are relatively low, although an interval of testosterone priming may be necessary. In all male primates, androgens increase sexual drive. When exposed to receptive females, male macaques increase their production of testosterone; in contrast, social subordination, and the stress associated with it, can reduce testosterone production (Rose et al., 1978). Stress reduces plasma testosterone in males and females via the hypothalamic–gonadal axis and also reduces, or even eliminates, mating behaviour.

Environmental exposures can influence reproductive function and mating behaviour. In some cases, these effects are mediated through visual or olfactory cues. For example, circadian rhythms influence the timing of the periovulatory surge of LH and the rate of ovulation. The LH surge tends to occur at night and in the morning (Seibel et al., 1982; Testart et al., 1982). The best evidence of seasonal variation in human reproduction is from studies in Alaskan Inuit, which show that seasonal changes in birth rates correspond to peaks in June and January (Ehrenkranz, 1983). Humans do not reproduce in a rigidly seasonal manner, possibly because they are less sensitive than other species to environmental cues or because they live in civilized or urbanized environments in which the impacts of environmental influences are attenuated (Van Vugt, 1990). Macaques breed seasonally in temperate environments but ovulate year-round when environmental conditions are maintained in a non-seasonal manner (Vandenbergh & Vessey, 1968; Van Vugt, 1990). However, macaques that are reared indoors and exposed to varying photoperiods still ovulate year-round. This suggests that humans no longer mate in a seasonal manner that reflects annual variation in photoperiods because of ontogenic and possibly evolutionary experience.

Hormonal control of mating behaviour is well documented in animals. In rats, estrogen and, to a lesser extent, progesterone control lordosis behaviour via the central nervous system (CNS). In female non-human primates, attractiveness and proceptivity change during the menstrual cycle or as a result of sex steroid administration. The effects of hormones on receptivity are unclear. It is assumed that steroid hormones influence behaviour in humans as they do in animals; however, it is difficult to differentiate the effects of social and other environmental factors from the effects of sex steroids on mating behaviour in humans.

Male mating behaviour has been studied predominantly in rodents as well as in other mammalian species. The male mating repertoire involves precopulatory behaviour, mounting, intromission, ejaculation and postejaculatory behaviour. The preoptic anterior hypothalamic area controls important aspects of male mating behaviour. Rhesus monkeys with bilateral lesions in this area do not attempt to copulate but can masturbate and achieve erections, indicating a deficit in mating behaviour towards the female, but no obvious neuroendocrine physiological compromise (Eisenberg, 1981).

3.6   Gamete transport

In most mammals, spermatozoa become motile while in the proximal cauda epididymis. The epididymis is also a reservoir for sperm. In addition, maturation of the spermatic plasma membrane in the epididymis involves physical and chemical alterations in the membrane lipids. Seminal and prostatic fluids are added to the semen during its passage through the male reproductive tract.

Human semen is deposited in the anterior vagina during coitus. There are usually between 20 and 120 million sperm per millilitre in human ejaculate (WHO, 1999). For fertilization to occur, sperm deposited in the vagina must travel to the fallopian tubes, and the ovum must be released from the ovary and transported within the fallopian tubes. Vaginal mucus protects the spermatozoa in the acidic vaginal environment from being ingested by macrophages. Spermatic movement through the cervix may continue for days, and most spermatozoa die during this manoeuvre. Prostaglandins in the semen stimulate uterine contractions that facilitate movement of spermatozoa through the uterus. Only a small proportion of deposited spermatozoa reach the site of fertilization in the mid-fallopian tube. Before ovulation, the vaginal mucus is thin and watery, allowing spermatozoa to pass more readily than the thicker mucus that forms after ovulation. Spermatozoan motility is necessary for movement up the female reproductive tract to the oviduct. Immotile spermatozoa are an easily detected cause of infertility in males. Another common cause of male infertility is spermatozoa that cannot penetrate the cervical mucus; this problem can be assessed to some extent *in vitro* (Eggert-Kruse et al., 1989).

Capacitation is the physiological change that makes spermatozoa capable of fertilization. While the sperm are in the male reproductive tract, capacitation is blocked by a decapacitation factor, but this factor is no longer active on sperm that have been deposited in the female reproductive tract. After capacitation, spermatozoa can demonstrate hyperactivated motility, undergo the acrosome reaction and bind with the zona pellucida of an unfertilized egg (Yanagimachi, 1970). Capacitation begins when spermatozoa are in the cervical mucus and continues until sequestration in the isthmus. Capacitation involves changes in intracellular ion concentrations (e.g., K^+, Na^+ and Ca^{2+}), increased metabolism, stabilization of disulfide bonds in nuclear proteins and removal of decapacitation factors from the plasma membrane.

At ovulation, the ovum, surrounded by the cumulus oophorus, is released from the ovary and moves down the fallopian tubes. As described above, ovulation follows a surge in LH, which causes luteinization of the granulosa cells of the follicle destined for ovulation. During ovulation, the oocyte enters the tubal lumen and is eventually moved to the site of fertilization. Since mating can occur at any time in the cycle in humans, the spermatozoa may be at the fallopian tubes at the time of ovulation, or the ovum may be at the fallopian tubes awaiting the arrival of the spermatozoa.

After fertilization, in the isthmus of the fallopian tubes, the zygote moves to the uterus for implantation. Prostaglandins, catecholamines, estrogen and progesterone stimulate contractions of the smooth muscle in the walls of the fallopian tubes, which move the zygote to the uterus.

3.7   Fertilization

Fertilization is the fusion of the sperm and ovum. The sperm head binds to the plasma membrane of the egg (oolemma), and the entire spermatozoon enters the cytoplasm of the ovum. Only capacitated spermatozoa with intact acrosomes can enter and pass through the cumulus oophorus. The acrosome is a membrane-bound, cap-like structure covering the anterior portion of the sperm nucleus. The acrosomal reaction is the release of materials that lyse the glycoprotein coat (zona pellucida) surrounding the ovum. This is necessary for fertilization to take place. Before undergoing the acrosomal reaction, sperm go through a type of hypermotility called hyperactivation. The hypermotility involves vigorous, whiplash beating of the tail and linear dashing movements. Hyperactivity appears to begin in the isthmus of the fallopian tubes and is thought to facilitate movement in the fluid of the oviduct (fallopian tubes) and to provide the power necessary to penetrate the cumulus oophorus and zona pellucida.

The acrosome reaction is the loss of the acrosomal and plasma membranes in the acrosome region and the release of acrosin, hyaluronidase and other enzymes that disperse the cumulus complex and allow the sperm to penetrate the zona pellucida. After capacitation and the acrosome reaction, sperm penetrate the extracellular cumulus matrix and bind with zona protein 3, a heavily glycosylated protein of the zona pellucida. The first segment of the sperm to make contact with the oolemma is usually the inner acrosomal membrane, followed by the postacrosomal region. The plasma membrane of the sperm attaches to microvilli on the oolemma. Sperm–egg fusion is apparent from reduced movement of the sperm tail (Yanagimachi, 1970, 1988; Takano et al., 1993). Once a sperm fuses with the egg membrane, the zona pellucida undergoes structural changes that form a physical barrier preventing additional sperm from entering the egg. After fusion with the sperm, the egg resumes meiosis, the second polar body is extruded and the male and female pronuclei fuse. Once the pronuclear envelopes of the sperm and egg have fused, the chromatin condenses, and the first mitotic division begins with the first cleavage. This first cleavage is the beginning of blastogenesis.

3.8   *In utero* development

3.8.1   *Blastogenesis*

Preimplantation development commences with a single cell and concludes with implantation of a late blastocyst. Preimplantation development has been well characterized and described in detail (Moore, 1988). The single-cell zygote progresses through two-, four- and eight-cell stages, during which the blastomeres are loosely attached to each other. Late in the eight-cell stage, the blastomeres become compact, and tight junctions form. The next cell division forms the 16-cell morula, characterized by inner cells that are surrounded by other blastomeres. By the 64-cell stage, the inner cells form the inner cell mass (ICM). The ICM forms the fetus, and the trophectoderm forms a connection with the uterus. Secretions from trophoblast cells form a blastocoele, and the ICM becomes located at one end of the cavity; the overlying cells are termed polar trophectoderm, and the rest are termed mural trophectoderm. All cell divisions up to this point are cleavage or reductive in nature. Because of this fact, the size of the embryo does not increase up to this point. In mammalian species, these cleavage events occur in the fallopian tube as the embryo is transported to the uterus, which takes approximately 7 days in humans and variable amounts of time in other mammals.

By the 8th day after fertilization, the trophectodermal cells are organized into two layers, an inner layer of mononucleated cells (cytotrophoblast) and an outer layer of larger, multinucleated cells that form the implantation syncytium (syncytiotrophoblast). The inner, mononucleated cells continue to form giant cells that are pushed progressively to the outer layers. The cells that make up the inner layer form the embryo, aggregate at one pole of the blastocyst and divide to form the bilaminar germ disc, with a layer of small cuboidal cells (hypoblasts) and a layer of high columnar cells (epiblasts).

3.8.2 Implantation

When the embryo arrives in the uterine cavity, the trophectoderm infiltrates the uterine epithelium by a poorly characterized mechanism. Several maternal and embryonic factors are crucial to implantation. These factors include colony stimulating factor, leukaemia inhibitory factor, interleukin-6 and several proteolytic enzymes. Before the placenta develops, the implanted embryo is nourished by histotrophic material from degradation of endometrial cells during implantation. The embryo is also nourished by secretions from endometrial glands and by the yolk sac; the latter persists for different time periods and plays different roles in different species.

The blastocyst implants into the maternal endometrial wall on about the 7th day of embryonic life. Trophoblastic cells attach to the uterine mucosa by apposition and adhesion. Under the influence of progesterone and estrogen, the uterine lumen closes, which brings the blastocyst into close contact with the endometrium. Adhesion of the trophoblast to the uterine epithelium occurs with increasing apposition and involves cell surface glycoproteins. The uterine epithelium is penetrated by syncytial growths on the trophoblast into the adjacent uterine epithelial cells. Subsequently, the trophoblastic membranes share junctional complexes and desmosomes with the uterine epithelial cells. The syncytial trophoblastic processes penetrate the basal lamina of endometrial blood vessels.

Decidualization of the endometrium occurs as a response to implantation. The decidualized endometrium is thickened due to proliferation of endometrial stromal cells, infiltration of inflammatory cells, increased vascular permeability, engorgement of blood vessels and oedema. Sustained exposure of the endometrium to both progesterone and estrogen is necessary for decidualization. Antiprogestins or high doses of estrogen disturb the estrogen/progesterone balance and inhibit decidualization and implantation.

3.8.3   Placentation

The placenta is a temporary organ that forms from the trophectoderm of the embryo and maternal cells. The fetal portion of the placenta develops from the chorionic sac, while the maternal portion arises from the endometrium. The placenta carries out a number of important functions, which include anchoring the developing fetus to the uterine wall, providing nutrients for the fetus and removing waste products. In addition, hormones are synthesized in the placenta, which maintain pregnancy and promote development of the fetus. Apart from its role in maternal–fetal interchange, the placenta is involved in metabolism and endocrine secretion. The placenta synthesizes glycogen, cholesterol and fatty acids early in gestation and produces large quantities of progestins and estrogens. The placental syncytioblast secretes hCG and human placental lactogen (hPL).

Gases, nutrients, hormones, electrolytes, antibodies and waste products are transported across the placenta. Many drugs and infectious agents can also cross the placenta. Maternal transfer of steroid hormones across the placenta is limited. When natural or synthetic steroid hormones do cross the placenta, developmental toxicity can result. Furthermore, hormones produced by the fetal placenta also play an important role in parturition.

In mammals, two distinct placentas, the yolk sac placenta and the chorioallantoic placenta, which develops during the first 40 days of development, are present early in development. Placentation involves complex vascular remodelling in both maternal and fetal circulation.

Vasculogenesis is regulated by several gene products, including vascular endothelial growth factors and the angiopoietins and their receptors (see Smith et al., 2000). The expression of these genes is regulated in a temporally and spatially ordered manner in the maternal–fetal interface, and they are principal mediators in the development of the normal placenta. Disruption of their function causes disturbances of implantation and vasculogenesis of the placenta.

3.8.3.1   Yolk sac placenta

In rodents, the yolk sac transports materials that are absorbed from the chorion and chorionic cavity before the allantoic (embryochorionic, fetoplacental) circulation is established. In humans, the yolk sac placenta functions in haematopoiesis, protein secretion and formation of the primordial germ cells. After the first trimester, the yolk sac becomes vestigial; by day 40 of gestation, the yolk sac is in the developing umbilical cord. The yolk sac provides nutrients to the developing fetus for approximately 92 days in the hamster, 10 days in mice, 12 days in the rat and 1 month in humans. In the rat and rabbit, the yolk sac nourishes the fetus until late in pregnancy, when it is separated from the gut. In rodents, the yolk sac placenta is the principal organ providing postimplantation nutrition to the embryo, and the chorioallantoic placenta is the site of attachment to the uterus. It is not until day 12 of gestation that the chorioallantoic placenta provides nutrients in the rodent.

3.8.3.2   Chorioallantoic placenta

The chorioallantoic placenta is the principal placenta in mammals, but the number of layers separating the maternal and fetal circulations and the shape of the layers vary. The fundamental unit of the mature placenta is the cotyledon, which is formed by a single placental disc in humans, rabbits and rats, but by two placental discs in monkeys. In humans, the villous tree transports materials between the maternal and fetal circulation. The villous tree is composed of fetal capillaries, associated endothelium, stromal cells and the macrophages known as Hofbauer cells. The trophoblast cells include the cytotrophoblast stem cells in one layer and a second layer of syncytiotrophoblast cells that secrete hCG and steroids early in pregnancy. Later in pregnancy, the syncytiotrophoblast produces large quantities of hPL. Extravillous trophoblast produces hPL early in gestation and proteolytic enzymes, resulting in the invasion of trophoblastic cells into the myometrium, replacing the endothelium in maternal blood vessels. Invasion and attachment of the trophectoderm are followed by the flow of blood in both the maternal and fetal circulations. The maternal blood is not in direct contact with the villous tissue until 10 weeks of gestation. In humans, embryochorionic circulation begins around 28–30 days of gestation. There is a gap of approximately 14 days between the establishment of the maternochorionic and embryochorionic circulation.

The placenta is essential for exchange of substances between the mother and the fetus. The fetal placenta develops from the chorionic sac, and the maternal placenta develops from the endometrium. By the end of the 3rd week, the primary chorionic villi develop, begin to branch and become surrounded by secondary chorionic villi. Blood vessels differentiate from spaces within the villi and become tertiary chorionic villi. Vessels in the chorion are connected to vessels in the embryo and to the heart primordia.

By the beginning of the embryonic period, oxygen and nutrients in the maternal blood diffuse through the walls of the villi into fetal vessels, and carbon dioxide and waste products diffuse from the fetal capillaries into the vessels of the maternal endometrium. During this period, the villi extend over the entire amniotic cavity. By the end of the embryonic period, maternal blood enters the vessels in the villi from endometrial arteries, while blood is carried away from the villi by endometrial veins. Fetal membranes form a barrier between fetal and maternal compartments. The fetal placenta is attached to the maternal placenta by the cytotrophoblastic shell, which is an extension of the cytotrophoblast through the syncytiotrophoblast. The villi from the cytotrophoblastic shell anchor the placenta to the endometrium. The villi from the syncytiotrophoblast are the main sites of exchange between maternal and fetal blood. By the 15th week, the decidua forms septa that project into the villi vessels. Syncytial cells cover the surfaces of the septa such that the maternal blood does not directly contact fetal tissue. The formation of septa compartmentalizes the placenta into cotyledons. In humans, the thin separation between maternal and fetal blood is called the haemochorial placentation.

3.8.3.3   Placental steroidogenesis

Both the cytotrophoblast and the syncytiotrophoblast synthesize peptide hormones, but only the syncytiotrophoblast produces steroid hormones. The placenta lacks certain steroidogenic enzymes and can not use acetate and cholesterol to produce progestins, androgens or estradiol. Therefore, the fetus converts androgens from the maternal circulation and fetal sources. The placental enzyme sulfatase removes the sulfate moiety from dehydroepiandrosterone sulfate (DHEAS) to form DHEA, which is then converted by 3β-hydroxysteroid dehydrogenase (3β-HSD) to the androgen androstenedione. Interconversion between androgens and estrogens is driven by 17β-HSDs. There are seven types of β-HSDs that differ in their substrate specificity and activity.

Estriol is also produced by another pathway in the syncytiotrophoblast cells of the placenta; DHEAS from fetal adrenal is converted to 16α-hydroxydehydroepiandrosterone sulfate in the fetal liver, followed by removal of the sulfated chain to produce 16α-hydroxy-dehydroepiandrosterone, which is then aromatized to estriol. Estriol is the predominant estrogen produced during pregnancy, and almost all of the estriol and estradiol produced by the placental syncytiotrophoblast enters the maternal circulation. By the 7th week of gestation, the placenta produces the majority of the estrogen in the maternal circulation.

In the placenta, there are 17β-HSDs that reduce androstenedione to testosterone (in rodents) and estrone to estradiol (in rodents and humans) and 17β-HSDs that promote the opposite activity, possibly protecting the fetus from highly active hormones (Peltoketo et al., 1999).

3.9   Embryogenesis

Detailed reviews of embryogenesis of all organ systems can be found elsewhere (Brown, 1994). Embryogenesis (and indeed all of development) is particularly sensitive to exogenous insult because it involves dynamic interactions between cells (or groups of cells) and products of gene expression that occur within a very limited window of time (termed a "critical period"). If the scheduled developmental events fail to happen during this critical period, an irreversible abnormality almost invariably results. Some of the deleterious effects that can occur during embryogenesis are spontaneous abortion, developmental abnormalities or latent changes that are not detected until later stages of development. A classic example of the latter situation occurred in pregnant women whose children were adversely affected when the drug diethylstilbestrol (DES) was given during pregnancy (Herbst et al., 1971; Arai et al., 1983).

The human embryo develops a bilaminar disc at about the 2nd week; a small cavity develops among the epiblastic cells and enlarges to become the amniotic cavity. The amnion is the fluid-filled membranous sac immediately surrounding the embryo/fetus. The epiblastic cells are the primordial forms for fetal mesoderm, endoderm and ectoderm. The yolk sac arises from cells of the cytotrophoblast that form a continuous membrane with the hypoblasts of the bilaminar germ disc and surround the initial blastocyst cavity, now called the exocoelomic cavity. The trophoblast gives rise to a layer of cells loosely arranged as the extraembryonic mesoderm around the amnion. Spaces in the syncytiotrophoblast are filled with a mixture of maternal blood from ruptured, engorged endometrial capillaries and secretions from eroded endometrial glands. The spaces in the syncytiotrophoblast fuse to form networks that are the primordial version of the intervillous spaces of the placenta. Maternal blood seeps into and out of the spaces, beginning the formation of the uteroplacental circulation. The cytotrophoblast produces extensions called the primary chorionic villi that penetrate the syncytiotrophoblast. The extraembryonic coelom divides the extraembryonic mesoderm into two layers. The extraembryonic mesoderm lines the trophoblast and covers the amnion. The extraembryonic somatic mesoderm and the trophoblast next to it are the chorion, and the extraembryonic cavity is now the chorionic cavity.

The first indication of cranial differentiation occurs when the hypoblasts at the junction of the amnion and yolk sac form the prochordal plate. The next series of embryonic events includes gastrulation, neurulation and formation of the major organ systems. The primitive streak appears in the bilaminar disc; from it, mesenchymal cells form the mesodermal layer between the epiblast and hypoblast, giving rise to the trilaminar embryo. The notochord develops from mesenchymal cells and moves to an area of the prochordal plate. Cells from the primitive streak migrate cranially to form the oropharyngeal membrane and the primitive cardiogenic area. The embryonic ectoderm, which is the epiblast of the bilaminar stage, surrounds the developing notochord to form the neural plate. The ectoderm of the neural plate (ultimately to form the brain and spinal cord) grows cranially until it reaches the oropharyngeal membrane. The neural plate invaginates along its central axis and forms the neural tube. The neural tube completely separates from the surface ectoderm, which gives rise to the epidermis of the skin. Some ectodermal cells of the neural tube migrate to each side of the neural tube and form irregular, flattened masses called neural crests. The neural crests give rise to the sensory ganglia of the spinal and cranial nerves (Stykova et al., 1998).

Because elements that will later form the CNS appear earlier than most other systems in the developmental process, disturbances of neurulation may result in severe abnormalities of the brain and spinal cord. Other ectodermal thickenings, the otic placode and lens placode, develop into the inner ear and lens, respectively. A series of meso-dermal blocks called somites form around the neural tube, and these somites give rise to the axial skeleton. The intraembryonic coelom appears in the lateral mesoderm and later divides into the pericardial, pleural and peritoneal cavities. The intermediate mesoderm forms the nephrogenic cord, which later becomes the kidneys.

Kidney development provides a useful example of the kinds of events that occur in the development of an organ. The kidney is formed through reciprocally inductive interactions between two tissues of dif-ferent embryonic origin, the epithelial ureteric bud and the mesenchy-mal metanephric blastema. The ureteric bud arises from the distal region of the mesonephric (Wolffian) duct and grows into an area of mesenchyme of the nephrogenic cord, the metanephric blastema, that is committed to form the kidney. The metanephric mesenchyme consists of paired masses of cells, about 5000 cells in each, at the level of the hindlimb buds. The ureteric bud must grow 200–300 µm to contact the blastema. Contact between bud and blastema occurs on day 11 in the mouse, on day 12 in the rat and at the end of the 4th week in the human. On contacting the metanephric blastema, the ureteric bud induces the mesenchyme to condense around the tip of the bud. The condensed mesenchyme epithelializes and forms a nephron. At the same time, the mesenchyme induces the ureteric bud to branch and stimulates further outgrowth. The new branches of the ureteric bud contact more of the blastema, inducing new condensation and nephron formation. This reciprocal induction occurs over and over, eventually forming all of the nephrons of the kidney.

The ureteric bud develops into the ureter, and the swelling at its end becomes the renal pelvis. The repeated branching of the ureteric bud results in the formation of the major and minor calyces (the large ducts that empty into the renal pelvis) and the system of collecting tubules. The two major calyces form from the first branching of the ureteric bud, around the end of the 6th week.

Studies using transgenic mice show that lack of the gene for the bone morphogenetic protein BMP-7 also results in the failure of the collecting duct tree to develop. However, BMP-7 is produced by the ureteric bud and metanephric mesenchyme, so it may be that the failure of the ureteric bud derivatives to develop is secondary to effects on other aspects of kidney development. The C-ros gene, responsible for the production of a tyrosine kinase, is also expressed in the ureteric bud and appears to be important for ureteric bud elongation and branching. C-ros appears to recognize a membrane-bound ligand, so it requires contact with the blastema to be activated. Branching can be inhibited *in vitro* by heparin, activin and TGF-beta 1. It is not known whether these are active *in vivo*.

A number of substances have been shown to induce the meta-nephric mesenchyme to differentiate. One obvious candidate signalling molecule is nerve growth factor (NGF). The NGF receptor is present transiently on the mesenchyme before and during nephrogenesis, and the treatment of ureteric bud/metanephric mesenchyme cultures with antisense oligonucleotides to NGF receptor blocks the induction (Sariola & Sainio, 1998). However, adding NGF to metanephric mesenchyme cultured alone does not induce differentiation, so the selectivity of the oligonucleotide treatment has been questioned. One line of evidence suggesting that NGF is important is the presence of nerve cells in the ureteric bud. The nerve cells appear to play an integral role in the induction process, as antibodies to ganglioside G3, a cell surface antigen on the nerve cells, blocks induction *in vitro*.

How these interactions alert the genome of the mesenchyme to start transcribing the elements necessary for differentiation into neph-rons is not known. However, the early events involve the expression of WT1, a transcription factor critical for early kidney development. WT1 was discovered in Wilms tumour, a relatively common paediatric tumour, affecting 1 in 10 000. Wilms tumour is characterized by uncontrolled proliferation of metanephric mesenchymal stem cells, along with incomplete or inappropriate differentiation of these cells. WT1 has four zinc fingers and four alternative splice forms that appear to be localized differently within the nucleus.

WT1 is present in the metanephric mesenchyme before induction and is upregulated during induction. Blocking induction stops the production of WT1. WT1 is expressed at high levels during the condensation of the mesenchyme and its transition to epithelium. Its expression diminishes thereafter, except in the podocyte layer of Bowman's capsule. WT1 knockout mice do not develop kidneys. The metanephric mesenchyme from these mice cannot be induced by wild-type inducers.

WT1 is also expressed in other tissues in the embryo that undergo the unusual mesenchyme-to-epithelium transition, the mesothelium and the primary sex cords. Knockout of WT1 also results in agenesis of the gonads. Thus, one possible function of WT1 is to initiate this transition. WT1 regulates the expression of IGF-II, the IGF-I receptor, platelet-derived growth factor A chain and the early growth response gene Egr-1. All four genes appear to play a role in nephrogenesis. IGF-II levels are very high in Wilms tumour. The roles of the other genes have not been worked out fully, but it is possible that IGF and Egr-1 are involved in an autoregulatory loop with WT1.

PAX-2 is a pattern formation gene expressed during early nephrogenesis. PAX-2 appears to maintain the proliferative state and is downregulated by WT1. PAX-2 knockouts have renal agenesis, also indicating an important role for this gene; however, its specific function has yet to be determined. One possibility is that PAX-2 may stimulate the upregulation of WT1 in the induced mesenchyme and in early condensates.

A number of small proteins, such as BMP-7, Wingless-Int (WNT) and fibroblast growth factor (FGF-2), are candidate molecules for metanephric mesenchyme induction. BMP-7 is produced in the right place, BMP-7 knockout leads to renal agenesis and antibodies to BMP-7 block nephrogenesis *in vitro*. However, it is produced by tissues that cannot induce nephrogenesis in a co-culture. This suggests that BMP-7 is necessary for most, but perhaps not the earliest, events in nephrogenesis. FGF-2 is produced by the ureteric bud and induces nephrogenesis in rat, but not mouse, mesenchyme. Another argument against it being the inducer is that it is produced by tissues that cannot produce nephrogenesis, including previously induced nephrons. Cells transfected with WNT-1 can induce nephrogenesis, but neither WNT-1 nor any other known WNT protein has been identified in the right tissues at the right time of development. More work is needed to sort out the contributions of these and other factors in mesenchymal induction.

It is worth mentioning the homeobox HOX gene family as having involvement in kidney development. A number of HOX genes are expressed in a graded pattern in the nephron, suggesting that they may play a role in establishing proximal–distal polarity. Knockout of both the HOX a11 and d11 genes results in complete or almost complete renal agenesis. However, loss of either gene by itself has little adverse effect, suggesting some redundancy of function. The precise role of HOX genes in kidney development has yet to be determined.

After induction, two events occur: condensation of the mesenchyme around the ureteric bud, and transformation of the mesenchyme into epithelium. In order for condensation into a comma-shaped mass to occur, there has to be induction of a critical mass of cells, not all of which appear to be in contact with the ureteric bud. There appears to be some short-range signalling in the mesenchyme involving the secreted glycoprotein WNT-4. Mice lacking WNT-4 fail to form pretubular aggregates (as do PAX-2 knockouts). There also appears to be migration of induced cells away from direct contact with the ureteric bud, often several cell diameters distant. This may permit uninduced cells to contact the ureteric bud.

Condensation appears to result from changes in the extracellular matrix, particularly the synthesis of syndecan, a glycoprotein. Condensation can be blocked *in vitro* by heparin or heparan sulfate, and over a 48-h culture period these glycans decrease nephrogenesis by over 90%. However, neither chondroitin sulfate nor hyaluronic acid had any effect on condensation, even though the latter is similar to heparan sulfate. Mice null for the gene for heparan sulfate 2-sulfotransferase are born without kidneys. Ureteric bud outgrowth and expression of early markers of differentiation in the mesenchyme are not affected by this mutation. However, condensation of the differentiating mesenchyme fails to take place, and subsequent renal development is blocked.

The transition from mesenchyme to epithelium involves biochemical changes in the cells and the extracellular matrix. N-CAM expression on cell surfaces disappears, replaced by L-CAM (uvomorulin). Vimentin, a characteristic cytoskeletal component of mesenchyme, disappears, and cytokeratin, characteristic of epithelia, appears. There is a decrease in collagen I extracellularly and an increase in the basement membrane components laminin and collagen IV.

The metanephric mesenchyme has an extremely high rate of proliferation. The metanephros doubles in size every 8 h during the first 5 days. In the prospective renal cortex, the expression of PCNA, a marker for S-phase, occurs in a majority of cells. The proliferation rate is slowed significantly in BMP-7 knockouts (described above) and BF-2 knockouts. BF-2 is a transcription factor in the medullary stroma. It is likely that it controls the synthesis of a soluble growth factor that stimulates mesenchyme proliferation, but the identity of that factor is unknown.

Despite the high rate of proliferation, there is also significant apoptosis in the kidney. Apoptosis is associated with three processes of kidney development. The first is during early nephron formation, perhaps as a way to get rid of cells that did not undergo the mesenchyme–epithelial transition. The second phase of apoptosis sculpts the glomeruli, and the third phase occurs later in the medulla and renal pelvis. Mice that overexpress p53 have excessive cell death and develop kidneys that are smaller than normal. Mice that are null for the bcl-2 gene have excessive apoptosis early in renal development, followed by hyperproliferation. This leads to the development of cystic kidneys.

Prior to the 3rd week, embryonic nutrition occurs by diffusion of maternal blood. At that point, development of the primitive blood and blood vessels begins in the extraembryonic mesoderm of the yolk sac. These cells differentiate into angioblasts that form cords and clusters, which in turn canalize. Cells in the periphery become flat and form the endothelium, whereas the inner cells give rise to the primitive blood cells. By fusion and continuous budding, the extraembryonic vessels that have contact with maternal circulation establish contact with vessels arising from the embryo proper. The mesenchymal cells surrounding the primitive endothelial cells differentiate to form the muscular and connective tissues of the vessel wall. The primitive heart is formed from mesenchymal cells in the cardiogenic area, similarly to the formation of the blood vessels.

The gastrointestinal tract is formed from the endodermal germ layer. The embryo folds cephalo-caudally and laterally to incorporate the endodermal layer into the body cavity. At the cephalic end, the buccopharyngeal membrane is the boundary of the foregut. The hindgut terminates at the cloacal membrane. By the end of the 8th week, tissues and organ systems have developed, and the major features of the external body form have developed. The ectodermal layer has given rise to primordial forms of the central and peripheral nervous systems and the sensory epithelium of the ear, nose, eye and epidermis. The ectodermal layer also gives rise to the mammary and pituitary glands and the enamel of the teeth. The mesoderm gives rise to the kidneys, cartilage, bone, connective tissue, muscle, heart, blood, lymph cells, gonads (ovaries and testes), genital ducts, serous membrane lining the body cavities (pericardial, pleural and peritoneal), spleen and cortex of the adrenal gland. The endoderm gives rise to the gastrointestinal and respiratory tracts, tonsils, thyroid, parathyroid, thymus, liver, pancreas and epithelial linings throughout the body.

The connection between the placenta and the embryo is maintained by the umbilical cord. A tubular extension of the embryonic hindgut called the allantois contains blood vessels that become the umbilical vein and arteries. The allantois itself extends from the umbilicus to the urinary bladder; as the fetus develops, it involutes, leaving a residual thick tube called the urachus, which persists throughout life as the median umbilical ligament. The umbilical cord develops from the connecting stalk of the allantois and the yolk sac stalk. The two are pushed together by the developing amniotic cavity as it obliterates the chorionic cavity.

Two important aspects of early development of the reproductive tract are that the fetal gonad is structurally indifferent in male and female embyros and that the fetal reproductive system can therefore develop as male or female. Thus, the first major step in development of the reproductive system is establishing gonadal sex. Sex of the embryo depends on whether the spermatozoon carries an X or Y chromosome, and sexual differentiation of the indifferent structures in the gonad is necessary to form the male or female reproductive tract. The SRY gene on the Y chromosome is needed for testicular differentiation. The primitive gonad differentiates around the 7th week of gestation. Other genes implicated in normal differentiation of the male reproductive tract include, but are not limited to, WT1, steroidogenic factor 1 (Parker et al., 1996), DAX-1, SOX-9 and a variety of homeobox genes (Lindsey & Wilkinson, 1996; Pellegrini et al., 1997). In the fetal gonad, the development of the Sertoli cells results in synthesis of MIS, which initiates the removal of female structures (Behringer, 1995). The Sertoli cells also control the normal development of the Leydig cells, resulting in testosterone synthesis and the development of the vas deferens, epididymis and seminal vesicles. In rodents, most of these events take place in the second half of pregnancy, whereas in the human fetus, most events occur during the first trimester of pregnancy.

3.10 Fetal development

The fetal period in humans extends from the 9th week of gestation until birth. The fetus grows rapidly, and many of the organ systems formed during embryogenesis mature and develop. At the beginning of the fetal period, the head is half as long as the whole fetus. As growth of the body proceeds rapidly, the relative length of the head diminishes. Primary ossification centres appear in the skeleton by 12 weeks, and the limbs develop further. The external genitalia of males and females appear similar until the 9th week, but are different by the 12th week. Urine starts to form between the 9th and 12th weeks. In early stages, the eyes have a lateral orientation, but by 16 weeks, the eyes come closer together. By the 17th week, growth slows, and by the 20th week, the fetus is covered in fine, downy lanugo hair. From weeks 21 to 25, the respiratory system develops rapidly. By 26 weeks, the eyes open, hair on the head and body is well developed and toenails appear. The quantity of body fat increases, and subcutaneous deposition makes the skin less wrinkled. The site of erythropoiesis shifts from the spleen to the bone marrow. At 36 weeks, the girth of the torso increases, and growth slows. In this interval, the male fetus grows more rapidly than the female, resulting in a greater weight at birth for males. In the male fetus, full descent of the testes into the scrotum should occur by the 38th week.

Male and female gonadal development is discussed in section 3.12.2.

Kidney development can be used again here to illustrate the kinds of events that occur during organ maturation, which takes place during fetal and postnatal development. While the induction of the organ and formation of its basic structure are initiated in the embryonic period, differentiation of the nephrons is not complete until term in humans, and not until the 2nd week postnatally in rodents.

Nephrons form as generations of ureteric bud branches contact increasingly more distal regions of the metanephric blastema. The loose mesenchyme of the blastema condenses (i.e., the cells come together, leaving very little extracellular space) around the tip of the bud. The condensed mesenchyme becomes comma-shaped, with the tail of the comma always pointing away from the adjacent duct of the ureteric bud. It is at this comma-shaped stage that the condensed mesenchyme changes into epithelium. Blood vessels invade the indentation between the tail and body of the comma; these vessels will develop into the glomerulus. The comma begins to grow another tail at the end closest to the ureteric bud, thus becoming S-shaped. The new tail will become the distal tubule of the nephron and fuse with the ureteric bud/collecting duct. The distal part of the S-shaped tubule differentiates into the loop of Henle, proximal tubule and Bowman's capsule. The tubule elongates as development proceeds. The podocyte layer of Bowman's capsule forms around the blood vessels of the glomerulus as they develop. Induction and differentiation of nephrons occur continuously through the 38th week of gestation in humans and for 10–12 days postnatally in rats and mice. There are approximately 1.5 million nephrons per kidney in humans, and 1000–2000 in mice.

After epithelialization and the formation of the S-shaped tubule, there is still much that needs to occur in order for the nephron to function. Cells destined to form the podocyte layer of the glomerulus flatten out and lose some of the markers that characterized their earlier transition to epithelium, including c-MYC, HOX-c9, LFB-1 and LFB-3, while keeping a high level of WT1. Expression of more classical mesenchymal markers such as vimentin takes place, but the cells also keep a number of epithelial proteins such as desmosomal components. The result is a tissue that is more organized than most connective tissue but leakier than most epithelium, the optimum design for urine filtration.

The rest of the S-shaped tubule retains its epithelial character and segments into proximal tubule, loop of Henle and distal tubule. The cells lose expression of WT1, PAX-2 and n-MYC. Capillaries grow into the cleft in Bowman's capsule. These apparently arise from blood vessels in response to angiogenic factors from the nephron. One such factor is VEGF, known to be secreted by early nephrons.

The kidney begins to function as soon as there are functional nephrons at the corticomedullary junction. Nephron development continues during this time in the periphery of the cortex. Production of urine starts at about the end of the 3rd month in humans and by gestation day 17 or 18 in rats. Urine production is not necessary for waste excretion from the fetus, as this is taken care of by the placenta. Urine production is necessary to maintain proper amniotic fluid volume. Fetuses without kidneys or with insufficient urine production have oligohydramnios, too little amniotic fluid. Oligohydramnios can lead to abnormal development by physically confining the fetus, sometimes resulting in amputation or deformation of limbs *in utero.*

Fetal urine is rich in serum proteins, as glomerular filtration begins before the podocyte layer of the glomerulus is mature. Although the proximal tubules have tight junctions and are capable of some endocytosis, there is insufficient capacity to resorb all of the filtered protein. The glomerular filtration barrier and proximal tubule resorption mature about 7 days after birth in the rat.

The ability to produce a concentrated urine also matures over time. In the rat, this function is not mature until 2–3 weeks after birth. This is due to the lengthening of the loops of Henle and to maturation of ion transport function. Sodium influx from the renal tubular lumen stimulates proximal tubule growth and upregulates the expression of Na^+K^+-ATPase, the major transporter of sodium in the kidney, in the basolateral membranes of the epithelium.

Fetal and postnatal maturation of the nervous system need special mention, because the nervous system is the organ system that requires the longest time to mature. Outgrowth of neuronal processes, formation and deletion of synaptic contacts and myelination take place over an extended period of time in humans and laboratory animals. This extended maturation makes the brain susceptible to environmental insult for a long period. For example, adverse neurobehavioural outcomes can occur from maternal alcoholism during the embryonic or fetal period. Endemic cretinism results from hypothyroid conditions (attributable to dietary iodine deficiency) during the fetal and early postnatal periods.

3.11 Gestation

Maintenance of pregnancy depends on a functioning placenta, intact fetal membranes and a quiescent maternal myometrium. The fetal membranes separate the fetus from the mother, protecting the immediate environment of the fetus without contributing to its body. The amniotic fluid is composed of secretions of the cells that line the amniotic cavity and fetal urine. The fetus swallows amniotic fluid during gestation, and the fluid is absorbed into the fetal circulation. Amniocentesis can identify characteristics of the fetus before parturition, and fetal sex can be determined from the desquamated cells. Hormones, including progesterone, are critical for maintaining the maternal myometrium in a quiescent state. Preterm labour is of great concern, but is exceedingly difficult to control.

3.12 Gametogenesis and gonadogenesis

3.12.1 Gamete development

In mammals, sex is determined genetically by the presence or absence of a Y chromosome. If the Y chromosome is absent, ovaries and female reproductive organs develop; if the Y chromosome is present, testicular androgens and MIS cause male organs to develop. In male and female fetuses, primordial germ cells divide mitotically in the yolk sac until gonadal differentiation, and primordial germ cells appear in the wall of the yolk sac at the 3rd week of fetal life. About 2 weeks later, the gonadal ridge appears, which is the earliest sign of gonadal development. The primordial germ cells progress into the gonadal ridge by amoeboid movement at about 6 weeks. The gonadal ridge grows and surrounds the primordial germ cells, and together they form three histological components: the surface epithelium, the primitive cords and the gonadal blastema, made up of primordial germ cells and mesenchymal cells. After the gonads start to differentiate, the primordial germ cells continue to divide; these are called oogonia in females and gonocytes in males. The oogonia are transformed to oocytes by the initiation of meiotic division during the 3rd to 9th months of fetal life. The oocytes are arrested in the diplotene stage of the first meiotic prophase until puberty. The spermatogonia do not enter meiosis until puberty.

3.12.2 Gonadal and genital development

The male gonads start to differentiate about 7 weeks after conception, with organization of the gonadal blastema into testicular cords and stroma. The testicular cords are composed of gonocytes and primitive Sertoli cells. By the 8th week, the stroma between the testicular cords differentiate into Leydig cells, which start to synthesize testosterone almost immediately. This androgen production stimulates differentiation and proliferation of Leydig cells. Testosterone stimulates the growth and differentiation of the mesonephric ducts (Wolffian ducts), leading to development of the epididymis, ductus deferens and the accessory glands of the male reproductive tract.

The Sertoli cells secrete MIS, which preempts development of the female upper reproductive tract. The Leydig cells produce androgens, and the appearance and involution of Leydig cells are controlled by hCG.

During embryogenesis, testicular cords grow in length with adjacent mesonephric ducts and become canalized to form the rete testis. The testicular end of the mesonephric duct differentiates into the epididymis, while the remaining portion becomes the ductus deferens. The mesonephric ducts adjacent to the primitive testes establish contact with the testicular tubules to form the efferent ducts. The portion of the mesonephric duct immediately distal to the efferent ducts becomes elongated and convoluted to form the epididymis. Seminal vesicles develop from the distal mesonephric duct. The terminal portion of the mesonephric duct between the seminal vesicles and urethra becomes the ejaculatory ducts and the ampullae of the vas deferens. The testicular cords are separated from the surface epithelium by the tunica albuginea; the septa grows from the tunica to divide the testis into wedge-shaped lobules. The testicles start to descend into the inguinal canal during the 6th month of fetal life and enter the scrotal swelling shortly before birth. The prostate gland develops from the urogenital sinus as a secretory tubuloalveolar gland and surrounds the urethra at the base of the bladder in the adult.

The female gonads start to differentiate later than male gonads. The gonadal blastema begins to differentiate into medullary cords and stroma in the 8th week of fetal life. The medullary cords degenerate and leave mainly connective tissue. The cortex of the early ovary is made up of oogonia and epithelium. By the 11th week of fetal life, interstitial connective tissues intersect the epithelium, leading to compartments containing single oocytes surrounded by a single layer of epithelial cells. These are the primordial follicles. The connective tissue of the ovaries is referred to as the ovarian stroma and determines the size of the ovary. The epithelium of the follicles becomes cuboidal, and stroma-derived cells make up the thecal layer around the primary follicles. The ovaries descend into the pelvis by the 12th week of fetal life. The paramesonephric duct differentiates in the female to form the oviduct (fallopian tubes), uterus and proximal vagina. The distal vagina develops from the urogenital sinus.

3.13 Parturition

During parturition in humans, the fetus, placenta and fetal membranes are expelled from the uterus. The mechanisms triggering parturition are poorly understood but appear to involve a complex interplay between maternal and fetal factors (Challis & Lye, 1994). The maternal neurohypophysis releases oxytocin, which causes uterine contractions. Parturition involves endocrine communication between several organ systems, including 1) the fetal hypothalamic–pituitary–adrenal axis; 2) changes in placental steroids and prostaglandins; 3) uterine responses to stimuli; 4) increasing numbers of coordinated contractions of the uterus; and 5) labour. Steroids from the placenta, the decidua and fetal membranes induce the myometrium of the uterus to become more responsive to factors such as prostaglandins and oxytocin. Progesterone levels drop and estrogen levels rise, possibly antagonizing the suppressive action of progesterone on the uterus and stimulating the contractile action of oxytocin. Local uterine production of prostaglandins maintains myometrial contractions throughout parturition.

3.14 Lactation

Lactation provides the newborn with all nutrients required for growth and development and antibodies that confer passive immunity.

However, breast-feeding has also been identified as a source of exposure to chemical contaminants (WHO, 1988). Despite the presence of chemical contaminants in breast milk, it is generally thought that the benefits of breast-feeding outweigh the risks of potential harm from exposure to chemicals. Milk production is regulated by several hormones, including growth hormone, prolactin, adrenal steroids, thyroid hormones, calcitonin, parathyroid hormone, insulin, glucagon, oxytocin and growth factors such as IGF and EGF. Synthetic estrogen, progesterone or androgen, alone or in combination, can inhibit lactation. Details of the mechanisms regulating lactogenesis are reviewed elsewhere (Tucker, 1994).

The mammary gland consists of the external nipple and the system of ducts from the alveoli to the skin surface. The alveoli do not fully develop until a female experiences pregnancy and lactation. Cortisol, insulin and placental lactogen contribute to alveolar development, but estrogen and progesterone are most important. The cells that line the alveoli synthesize milk, and they are surrounded by a layer of myo-epithelial cells that eject the milk.

The mammary glands are essentially the same in males and females until puberty, when estrogen in females stimulates growth of the duct system, accumulation of fat cells and external development of breasts. Progesterone further stimulates development of the ducts. During pregnancy, estrogen and progesterone cause the ductal system of the mammary gland to branch and the alveolar cells to proliferate. In late pregnancy, milk secretion and letdown begin. The hormones involved that maintain lactation include ACTH, thyroxine, thyrotrophin releasing hormone and growth hormone. During lactation, the myoepithelial cells contract in response to suckling-induced oxytocin secretion from the posterior pituitary gland.

3.15 Maturation (postnatal)

The neonate grows rapidly after birth, organ and tissue systems increasing in size and fat deposition continuing. By 1 year after birth, human infants are 3 times their birth weight, and the rate of growth gradually decreases until puberty. An increase in the rate of body growth occurs again at puberty.

Human development lasts for an extended period of time. This pattern is related to delayed development in non-human primates, which leads to larger brain size and lower fecundity than in other species. Human size is dimorphic (males larger than females) starting at birth, and the dimorphism becomes more pronounced at adolescence. Males grow faster and for a longer period due to the delayed closure of epiphysial growth plates. Human body size is likely to be programmed by genetic factors, but a wide range of external and internal influences can affect adult body size.

During the first 6 months after birth, the H-P-G axis of infants is activated transiently, and surges of GnRH and pituitary gonadotrophin are secreted with increasing frequency. In males, the activity of the H-P-G axis increases the number of Sertoli cells and gonocytes and stimulates progression of gonocytes to spermatogonia. The H-P-G activity also causes transient secretion of testosterone by Leydig cells. This is critical for reproductive development, because it is a determinant of the maximum capacity for sperm production in the adult male.

Although the reproductive system appears to be functionally inactive in the neonate, infant and human child, evidence suggests that it is structurally and sexually mature and capable of functioning, but restrained by CNS inhibition. Possible CNS mechanisms for such repression are opioid inhibition of the GnRH pulse generator system or disconnection of GnRH neurons from catecholaminergic stimulation. The trigger for puberty remains elusive, but it is likely to involve the gonadal steroids estradiol and testosterone. Hypothalamic and pituitary sensitivity to the negative feedback effects of gonadal steroids decrease during the peripubertal period. Thus, higher levels of gonadal steroids are required to inhibit pituitary gonadotrophin secretion during this period.

The adolescent stage begins at puberty, when the capacity to reproduce is acquired. The timing of puberty is not well understood, but activation of the GnRH pulse generator is a key step in the process. The GnRH pulse generator system remains relatively quiescent during prepubertal years, but becomes active during the peripubertal period and attains the adult pulse frequency of one pulse every 45–90 min at puberty. External factors such as stress, weight loss and illness can disrupt the GnRH pulse generator system. Environmental contaminants can also affect sexual maturation, indicating that development of the H-P-G axis is sensitive to exogenous chemicals.

3.16 Reproductive senescence

In women, fertility declines around 35 years of age and continues to decline until the last menstrual cycle or menopause, which occurs at a mean age of 50. Preceding menopause, menstrual cycles become progressively longer and irregular and may be anovulatory. Circulating levels of estradiol during the perimenopausal period are lower, and serum LH and FSH levels are elevated. The principal cause of menopause is the loss of primordial follicles. Thus, variability in the onset of human menopause may be related to, among other factors, the number of follicles at menarche and different rates of follicle loss. Factors that affect the age of menopause include age of menarche, oral contraceptive use, weight loss, illness, stress and cigarette smoking. The role of environmental pollutants in ovarian failure and menopause is unknown, although it is plausible that long-term exposure to chemical contaminants could decrease the age of menopause onset (see chapter 4).

In contrast to women, men do not experience a sudden loss of fertility as they age, but circulating testosterone level and libido decline from approximately 40 years of age onwards (Gray et al., 1991; Vermeulen, 1993). Leydig cell function and the circulating level of testosterone are reduced in elderly men. These changes are associated with a decline in the number of Leydig cells and steroid synthesis. Furthermore, there is an age-related increase in the circulating level of FSH that is probably related to the decline in Sertoli cell function and decreased inhibin B production. In general, semen quality gradually declines with age, with semen of older men showing decreased sperm count and lower sperm motility.

3.17 Summary

Reproductive development and function depend on endocrine communication throughout the mammalian life cycle. Protein and steroid hormones, growth factors and other signalling molecules affect gene expression and protein synthesis in target cells of different tissues. In particular, fetal development, development of the reproductive tract, gametogenesis and gamete release are regulated by many hormonal signals that must be delivered at the appropriate level and at the correct moment during development. It is likely that the developing fetus is more sensitive to the effects of environmental pollutants than the adult; however, these effects *in utero* may not be manifested until adulthood is reached. Further characterization of the molecular mechanisms regulating normal development and reproduction is critical to our understanding of the disruptive effects of exogenous chemicals on these functions. Chapters 4 and 5 of this document are a detailed description of the methods used to evaluate reproductive and developmental toxicity resulting from chemical exposure. Chapter 6 extends this discussion to the area of human risk assessment for reproductive health in relation to environmental exposure.

4. EVALUATION OF ALTERED SEXUAL FUNCTION AND FERTILITY

4.1 Introduction

The purpose of this chapter is to review the methods that are currently in use to evaluate sexual function and fertility. Sexual function and fertility are complex reproductive functions that can be affected by environmental exposures. Reproductive disorders include spontaneous abortions, impaired spermatogenesis, menstrual disorders, impotence, early menopause and others. Any disturbance in the integrity of the reproductive system can affect these functions.

It is important to consider both *in vitro* and *in vivo* studies for evaluation of altered sexual function and fertility. *In vivo* studies are the primary basis for such reproductive toxicity testing, but *in vitro* studies (e.g., detailed studies on receptor interactions) that can provide a mechanistic explanation for the adverse effects observed *in vivo* are also useful.

For information on statutes and guidelines relevant to sexual function and fertility testing, the reader is referred to the references cited in chapter 2.

4.2 Experimental data

4.2.1 *In vivo experimental data*

4.2.1.1 *Introduction*

Laboratory rodents are the animal models most commonly used to identify hazards in reproductive toxicity. Rodents are used because they are small animals, the assay cost is moderate and there is a large database of toxicology information on these species (e.g., dose–response, metabolism, kinetics, etc.). The rat has proven to be a good model for human reproductive hazard evaluation (Francis et al., 1990).

Table 1. Selected indices of reproductive function[a]

Index	Calculation
Mating	$\dfrac{\text{Number of males or females mating}}{\text{Number of males or females cohabited}} \times 100$
Fertility	$\dfrac{\text{Number of cohabited females becoming pregnant}}{\text{Number of non-pregnant couples cohabited}} \times 100$
Gestation (pregnancy)	$\dfrac{\text{Number of females delivering live young}}{\text{Number of females with evidence of pregnancy}} \times 100$
Live birth	$\dfrac{\text{Number of live offspring}}{\text{Number of offspring delivered}} \times 100$ (on a litter basis)
4-day survival (viability)	$\dfrac{\text{Number of live offspring at p.n.}^{b}\text{ day 4}}{\text{Number of live offspring delivered}} \times 100$ (on a litter basis)
Lactation (weaning)	$\dfrac{\text{Number of live offspring at p.n. day 21}}{\text{Number of live offspring born}^{c}} \times 100$
Sex ratio	$\dfrac{\text{Number of male offspring}}{\text{Number of female offspring}} \times 100$

[a] Modified from US EPA (1998a).
[b] p.n. = postnatal.
[c] If litters are standardized at postnatal day 4 (or other times after birth), use number of offspring left after standardization. A number of post-birth indices may also be calculated on a litter basis.

2.1.2 General evaluation of sexual function and fertility

Table 1 lists a number of general indices of reproductive function. The mating index and fertility index are most useful when treatment begins prior to mating or implantation; in cases where treatment does not begin until after fertilization, however, they may indicate the general fertility of the stock of animals used. The gestation index and live birth index indicate the viability of young at birth, while the 4-day survival index and lactation index indicate the viability of pups to weaning.

Other measures include changes in gestation length and duration of parturition, which may indicate an effect on the process of parturition or alterations in *in utero* growth of the fetuses. Change in gestation length should be considered in any postnatal evaluation of pup body weights or other functional effects that depend on developmental stage, since pup weight increases at a different rate *in utero* and after birth.

Fertility assessment in test animals has limited sensitivity as a measure of reproductive injury, because, unlike humans, males of most test species produce sperm in excess of the minimum requirements for fertility. In addition, test animals can undergo multiple matings (Amann, 1981; Working, 1988; Chapin & Heindel, 1993). In some strains of rats and mice, production of sperm can be reduced by 90% or more without compromising fertility (Aafjes et al., 1980; Meistrich, 1982; Working, 1988); in human males, less severe reduction in sperm production can cause reduced fertility. Thus, measurement of change in sperm count or fertility in laboratory rodents may be insufficient to assess reproductive health risk in humans. Other animal models may be more suitable for assessing fertility (Chapin et al., 1998). However, it should not be assumed that a reduction in sperm count (i.e., <90%) will have no effect on fertility in rodents (Wine et al., 1997).

4.2.1.3   *Evaluation of male-specific end-points of sexual function and fertility*

Table 2 lists several common specific end-points that can be evaluated as measures of male sexual function and fertility, and these are discussed below. Developmental effects are discussed in chapter 5.

Table 2. Common male-specific end-points of sexual function and fertility[a]

End-point	Examples
Organ weights	Testes, epididymides, seminal vesicles, prostate, pituitary
Histopathology	Testes, epididymides, seminal vesicles, prostate, pituitary
Sperm evaluation[b,c]	Sperm number (count, concentration), quality (morphology, motility), chromosomal defects
Hormone levels[b]	LH, FSH, testosterone, estrogen, prolactin, inhibin B
Sexual behaviour	Mounts, intromissions, ejaculations
Developmental effects[d]	Testis descent,[b] preputial separation, sperm production,[b] anogenital distance, structure of external genitalia[b]

[a]   Modified from US EPA (1998a).
[b]   End-points that can be evaluated relatively easily in humans.
[c]   End-points currently being developed include aneuploidy and partial duplications, deletions and rearrangements.
[d]   See chapter 5.

1)   Organ weights

Absolute and relative (i.e., adjusted for body weight) organ weights should be considered, because a decrease in absolute weight may occur that is not necessarily related to a reduction in body weight gain. A significant increase or decrease in testis weight can indicate an adverse effect, but can be due to processes other than seminiferous tubular damage, such as oedema, inflammation, cellular infiltration, Leydig cell hyperplasia or fluid accumulation due to blocked efferent ducts (Hess, 1990; Nakai et al., 1993).

Pituitary gland weight can be an indicator of the reproductive status of the animal. However, the pituitary regulates a variety of physiological functions, including some that are separate from reproduction, and is composed of several cell types. If weight changes are observed, gonadotroph-specific histopathological evaluation may be useful to determine which cell types are affected. The weights of the prostate and seminal vesicle are androgen dependent and may reflect change in an animal's endocrine status or testicular function.

Changes in male reproductive organ weight could also justify additional studies on the reproductive toxicity of an agent. However, significant change in other important end-points related to reproductive function may not be accompanied by a change in organ weight. Therefore, it is insufficient to evaluate organ weight alone to assess reproductive toxicity of an agent, as other end-points may be more sensitive indicators.

2)   Histopathology

Histopathology on reproductive tissues is valuable for male reproductive toxicity assessment. Histological evaluations can be especially useful because they are a relatively sensitive indicator of damage and they provide information on toxicity from a variety of protocols. In addition, histological data can provide information on site (including target cells) and extent of toxicity after short-term testing and can also indicate the potential for recovery. The quality of histological analyses of spermatogenesis is improved by proper fixation and embedding of testicular tissue (Russel et al., 1990; Chapin & Heindel, 1993; Hess & Moore, 1993). Several approaches for qualitative or quantitative assessment of testicular tissue are available that can assist in the identification of less obvious lesions that may accompany lower-dose exposures (Hess, 1990; Russel et al., 1990). Significant dose-related increases in histopathological damage of any of the male reproductive organs should be considered an adverse reproductive effect. Significant histopathological damage in the pituitary should be considered an adverse effect but should involve gonadotrophin- or prolactin-producing cells to be considered a reproductive effect. The absence of histopathological effects may not be sufficient evidence to indicate no male reproductive system toxicity.

Morphometric and stereological research methods are valuable quantitative tools for toxicological studies. However, these methods can be very labour intensive and therefore are infrequently used for toxicity evaluation studies. Computerized image analysis may solve some of these problems in the future. Other automated quantitative methods, such as flow cytometry, have also been used (Kangasniemi et al., 1990; Toppari et al., 1990). However, these are not routine techniques and are not incorporated in any testing guidelines at present.

3)   Sperm evaluation

Sperm evaluations routinely include data on sperm number, morphology and motility (Berman et al., 1996). Testicular spermatid count or cauda epididymal weight are other useful measures of sperm production, but no surrogate measures are adequate to evaluate sperm morphology or motility. A number of other indices of sperm function have been employed (e.g., sperm–zona interactions, acrosome reaction, sperm swelling studies), but these have been of limited utility and infrequently used and have not been incorporated into any testing guidelines.

In test species, sperm number or sperm concentration can be evaluated in ejaculated, epididymal or testicular samples (Seed et al., 1996), but ejaculates can be obtained readily only from rabbits or dogs or from the reproductive tracts of mated females in rodents (Zenick et al., 1984). In humans, sperm production is usually evaluated in ejaculates, but can also be evaluated from spermatid counts or quantitative histology using testicular biopsy tissue, if available (Wyrobek, 1982, 1984).

Internationally accepted guidelines for analysing human semen have been established by WHO (1999). Similar principles can be followed for analysis of sperm from domestic animals (Amann, 1970). Efficiency of spermatogenesis can be evaluated by measuring DSP and DSP rate (Amann, 1970; Berendtson, 1977). Testes are homogenized or sonicated, and homogenization/sonication-resistant spermatids are counted in a haemocytometer. The results are expressed per testis or per gram of testis. DSP rate can be calculated on the basis of the kinetics of spermatogenesis, i.e., the length of the spermiogenic period when spermatids have compact, sonication-resistant nuclei. This time depends on the species and strain of animal. Sperm number can also be measured from epididymal homogenates. The epididymis is usually divided into distinct regions before homogenization, and the cauda is used for analysis of sperm motility. Computer-assisted videomicroscopy can be used to improve the objectivity of the assessment of sperm motility (Working & Hurtt, 1987; Slott et al., 1991), and videotapes (or digitized images) are useful means to store data. Sperm morphology can also be assessed by staining smears of epididymal spermatozoa with eosin Y (Wyrobek et al., 1983). Abnormalities of the head, midpiece, principal piece and tail can be recorded. Epididymal transit time is the number of days that spermatozoa stay in this organ, and this can be estimated from the ratio of the sperm counts in the testis and epididymis. Total cauda epididymal sperm count, percentage of progressively motile sperm, percentage of morphologically normal sperm and percentage of sperm with each abnormality are included in the US EPA testing guidelines (US EPA, 1998a) and the updated OECD Test Guidelines 414 (OECD, 2001a) and 416 (OECD, 2001b).

The number of sperm in an ejaculate is influenced by several variables, including the length of abstinence and the ability to obtain the entire ejaculate. Intra- and interindividual variability are often high, but less variability is observed in ejaculates collected at regular intervals from the same male (Williams et al., 1990). Because sperm contribute to epididymal weight in experimental animals, expression of results as a ratio of sperm counts to epididymal weight may actually mask a decline in sperm number, and absolute sperm counts can improve resolution.

Sperm production can be evaluated by counting spermatids as a substitute for quantitative histological analysis (Russel et al., 1990); however, this analysis may not detect the effects of a short-term exposure. Spermatid counts can also help detect a decrease in testicular sperm production; however, this index reflects only the integrity of spermatogenic processes within the testes.

Sperm morphology can be evaluated in cauda epididymal, vas deferens or ejaculated samples. Sperm head morphology has frequently been reported in toxicology studies because of the suggested correlation between mutagenicity and abnormal sperm morphology (Wyrobek et al., 1983). Methodologies, such as *in situ* hybridization, can be adapted to detect several types of chromosomal defects in human sperm and examine paternally transmitted genetic defects (Sloter et al., 2000). However, not every mutagen induces sperm head abnormalities, and some non-mutagenic chemicals alter sperm head morphology. Sperm morphology is one of the least variable sperm characteristics in normal individuals, which may enhance its usefulness as an indicator of spermatotoxic events (Zenick et al., 1984). However, the reproductive implications of abnormal sperm morphology need to be delineated more fully. The majority of studies in test species and humans suggest that abnormally shaped sperm may not reach the oviduct or participate in fertilization (Porcelli et al., 1984). The implication is that abnormal sperm are likely to reduce fertility.

Sperm motility can be selectively affected by chemicals (e.g., epichlorohydrin) that reduce fertility. Studies have examined rat sperm motility as a reproductive end-point (Morrissey et al., 1988a, 1988b; Toth et al., 1991a, 1991b), and sperm motility assessments are an integral part of some reproductive toxicity test guidelines (Gray et al., 1988; Morrissey et al., 1988a, 1988b, 1989; US EPA, 1998a). Motility estimates may be obtained on ejaculated, vas deferens or cauda epididymal samples, and standardized methods for both manual and automated assessments are available (Chapin et al., 1992). In studies using automated technology, chemically induced alterations in sperm motion were detected and related to the fertility of the exposed animals (Toth et al., 1991a, 1991b; Slott et al., 1995). These preliminary studies indicate that significant reductions in sperm velocity are associated with infertility, even when the percentage of motile sperm is not affected.

Changes in spermatogenesis and sperm maturation have been related to fertility in several test species, but infertility cannot be reliably predicted from these data. This is in part due to the fact that fertility is determined by sperm number and quality. If sperm quality is high, then sperm number must be substantially reduced before fertility is affected. In humans, the mean sperm count for fertile men is higher than the mean for infertile men, but the distributions of sperm counts for fertile and infertile men overlap (Meistrich & Brown, 1983); nevertheless, fertility is likely to be impaired when sperm count drops below 20 million per millilitre (WHO, 1999). Others (Bonde et al., 1998a, 1998b) have suggested that this level may be more like 40 million per millilitre. Similarly, if sperm number is normal in rodents, a relatively large effect on sperm motility is required before fertility is affected. Thus, it is important to assess several sperm measures, reproductive organ histopathology and fertility to properly assess reproductive toxicity. Chemical testicular toxicants can also interfere with spematozoa in the male excurrent ducts. Only a few studies have assessed the effects of environmental chemicals on seminal chemistry and accessory glands (Contreras & Bustos-Obregõn, 1996; Contreras et al., 1999). Specific information about reproductive organ and gamete function can then be used to evaluate the extent of injury and the probable site of toxicity in the reproductive system.

4)   Hormone levels

The male reproductive system can be affected adversely by disruption of the normal endocrine balance. In adults, effects that interfere with normal concentrations or action of LH and/or FSH can decrease or abolish spermatogenesis, affect secondary sex organ (e.g., epididymis) and accessory sex gland (e.g., prostate, seminal vesicle) function and impair sexual behaviour (Sharpe, 1994). Significant alterations in circulating levels of testosterone, LH or FSH may indicate pituitary or gonadal injury and may be related to alterations in spermatogenesis, sperm maturation, mating ability or fertility. Furthermore, such hormonal effects can help understanding of the site or mechanism of toxicant action, especially for short-term exposures.

5)   Sexual behaviour

Sexual behaviour reflects complex neural, endocrine and reproductive organ interactions and can be disrupted by a variety of toxic agents, diseases and pathological conditions. For example, neurotoxic agents that have agonist or antagonist androgenic or estrogenic properties can affect sexual behaviour. Interference with sexual behaviour in either sex by environmental agents represents a potentially significant human reproductive problem, and significant alteration in sexual behaviour should be considered an adverse effect.

Most information comes from studies on effects of drugs on sexual behaviour in humans. Data on sexual behaviour are usually not available from studies of human populations that were exposed occupationally or environmentally to potentially toxic agents, nor are such data obtained routinely in studies of environmental agents with test species. Although the functional components of sexual performance can be quantified in most test species, no direct evaluation of this behaviour is done in most breeding studies. Rather, copulatory plugs or sperm-positive vaginal lavages are taken as evidence of sexual receptivity and successful mating. However, these markers do not demonstrate whether male performance resulted in adequate sexual stimulation of the female to facilitate transport of the sperm along the female reproductive tract to ensure fertilization. In the male rat, measures include latency periods to first mount, mount with intromission and first ejaculation, number of mounts with intromission to ejaculation and the postejaculatory interval (Beach, 1979; Chubb, 1993).

4.2.1.4   *Evaluation of female-specific end-points of sexual function and fertility*

A variety of measures have been used to evaluate effects on the female reproductive system in animal toxicity studies (Mattison & Thomford, 1989; McLachlan & Newbold, 1989). Reproductive toxicity can be evaluated in a comprehensive manner in females, including identification of target organs and, in some cases, a mechanistic understanding of the effects of an agent. Table 3 lists several end-points of sexual function and fertility that can be evaluated in females. The reproductive life cycle of the female is divided into fetal, prepubertal, cycling adult, pregnant, lactating and senescent phases. The reproductive status of the female should be known when measurements are made, especially at necropsy, for proper detection and interpretation of reproductive effects.

1)   Organ weights and histopathology

Significant change in ovary weight should be considered an indication of female reproductive toxicity. In the rat, ovarian weight does not normally fluctuate during the estrous cycle. However, even if

Table 3. Common female-specific end-points of sexual function and fertility[a]

End-point	Examples
Organ weights	Ovary, uterus, vagina, pituitary
Histopathology	Ovary, uterus, vagina, pituitary, oviduct, mammary gland
Estrous (menstrual) cycle[b]	Vaginal smear cytology
Hormone levels[b]	LH, FSH, estrogens, progesterone, prolactin
Sexual behaviour	Lordosis, time to mating, vaginal plugs or sperm
Lactation	Milk quantity, quality, maternal behaviour, pup suckling behaviour, offspring growth
Development[c]	Normality of external genitalia, vaginal opening, vaginal smear cytology, onset of estrous behaviour (menstruation)
Senescence	Vaginal smear cytology, ovarian histology (menopause)

[a] Modified from US EPA (1998a).
[b] End-points that can be evaluated relatively easily in humans.
[c] See chapter 5.

ovary weight does not change, toxicity can still be evident by other measures, such as histological evaluation of the ovary.

Histological evaluation should be carried out on the three major compartments of the ovary (i.e., follicular, luteal and interstitial), the epithelial capsule and ovarian stroma. Methods are available to determine the number of follicles and their stages of maturation (Smith et al., 1991). These techniques may be useful to determine if the pool of primordial follicles is depleted or their subsequent development or recruitment for ovulation is altered by exposure to toxic agents (Smith et al., 1991). Significant histological change in any of the following features should be considered adverse: incidence of follicular atresia; number of primary follicles; number or life span of corpora lutea; and folliculogenesis or luteinization, including cystic follicles, luteinized follicles and frequency of ovulation.

An alteration in the weight of the uterus can indicate reproductive toxicity. Compounds that inhibit steroidogenesis and cyclicity can dramatically reduce the weight of the uterus so that it appears atrophic and small. However, uterine weight fluctuates 3- to 4-fold during the estrous cycle, peaking at proestrus, when it is filled with fluid and distended in response to secreted estrogen. Other indicators of uterine growth include epithelial height and lactoferrin production in mice.

Reproductive toxicity can also be assessed in pregnant or postpartum animals. In such cases, the number of implantation sites, live pups and resorptions should be counted. Gravid uterine weight will vary with each of these factors. Pre- and postimplantation loss are calculated from this information and the corpus luteum count. Gravid uterine weight is sometimes subtracted from total pregnancy weight gain to determine whether changes are due to intrauterine effects or toxicity to the dam.

The histological appearance of the uterus fluctuates with stage of the estrous cycle and pregnancy. The uterine endometrium is sensitive to estrogens and progestagens (Warren et al., 1967), and extended treatment with these compounds leads to hypertrophy and hyperplasia. Conversely, inhibition of ovarian activity and reduced steroid secretion results in endometrial hypoplasia and atrophy, as well as altered vaginal smear cytology. The following effects on the uterus may be considered adverse: infantile or malformed uterus or cervix, decreased or increased uterine weight, endometrial hyperplasia, hypoplasia or aplasia and decreased number of implantation sites.

Typically, the oviducts are not weighed or examined histologically in tests for reproductive toxicity. However, the following changes, if reported, should be considered adverse: hypoplasia of the oviducts and loss of cilia, resulting most commonly from lack of estrogen stimulation (may not be recognized until after puberty); hyperplasia of the oviductal epithelium, resulting from prolonged estrogenic stimulation; or developmental anomalies, including agenesis, segmental aplasia and hypoplasia.

Vaginal weight change should parallel uterine weight change during the estrous cycle, although the magnitude of the vaginal change is smaller. In rodents, cytological change in the vaginal epithelium (observed in vaginal smears) can identify stages of the estrous cycle. Altered cyclicity such as persistent estrus or diestrus can also be detected by vaginal smears. The vaginal smear pattern can also identify conditions that would delay or preclude fertility or affect sexual behaviour. Histological alterations that can be observed include aplasia, hypoplasia and hyperplasia of the vaginal epithelial cell lining. Developmental changes may result in agenesis, hypoplasia and dysgenesis of the vagina. Hypoplasia of the vagina can be concomitant with hyperplasia of the external genitalia, thus altering the anogenital distance. The opening of the vaginal orifice at puberty provides a simple and useful developmental marker. The following effects on the vagina can be considered to be adverse: infantile or malformed vagina or vulva, masculinized vulva or increased anogenital distance, vaginal hypoplasia or aplasia, altered timing of vaginal opening and abnormal vaginal smear cytology.

Alterations in weight of the pituitary gland can be considered an adverse effect in females. Pituitary weight increases normally with age, as well as during pregnancy and lactation. Change in pituitary weight can also occur as a consequence of chemical stimulation. Increased pituitary weight often precedes tumour formation, particularly in response to treatment with estrogenic compounds. Increased pituitary size associated with estrogen treatment can be accompanied by hyperprolactinaemia and a persistent vaginal cornified smear pattern. Decreased pituitary weight is less common but can result from decreased estrogenic stimulation (Cooper et al., 1989). Significant histopathological damage in the pituitary should be considered an adverse effect, as discussed above for males, but should involve cells that produce gonadotrophin or prolactin to be called a reproductive effect.

Mammary gland size and histology change dramatically prior to and at the onset of parturition and can be adversely affected by toxic agents. Some chemicals and drugs reduce milk availability and quality. Perinatal exposure to steroid hormones and other chemicals can alter mammary gland morphology and tumour potential in adulthood. Cleared and stained whole mounts of the mammary gland can be examined histologically. Altered DNA, RNA or lipid content can indicate toxicity to the mammary gland.

2)   Estrous cycle

The events of the estrous cycle can be used as an indicator of reproductive neuroendocrine and ovarian function in the non-pregnant female. Hormonal, histological and morphological measurements can also be interpreted relative to stage of the cycle and can be used to monitor the status of mated females. With cycling females, vaginal smear cytology should be examined daily for at least three normal estrous cycles prior to treatment, after onset of treatment and before necropsy (Kimmel et al., 1995). Daily vaginal smear data from rodents can be used to evaluate the following: (1) cycle length, (2) occurrence or persistence of estrus, (3) duration or persistence of diestrus, (4) incidence of spontaneous pseudopregnancy, (5) pregnancy versus pseudopregnancy (based on the number of days the smear remains leukocytic), (6) presence of sperm in the vagina as an indication of mating and (7) acyclicity as an indication of reproductive senescence. The technique can also detect reproductive senescence in rodents (LeFevre & McClintock, 1988). Evidence of dose-related disruptions in the estrous cycle, including abnormal cycle length or pattern or failure to ovulate, should be considered an adverse effect.

The corpus luteum arises from the ruptured follicle and secretes progesterone, which has an important role in the estrous or menstrual cycle. Luteal progesterone is also required to maintain early pregnancy in most mammalian species, including humans (Csapo & Pulkkinen, 1978). Therefore, establishment and maintenance of normal corpora lutea are essential for normal reproductive function. However, with the exception of evaluations to establish their presence or absence, these structures are not evaluated in routine testing. Increased rates of follicular atresia and oocyte toxicity may lead to premature menopause in humans. Altered follicular development, failure to ovulate or altered corpus luteum formation and function can disrupt cyclicity, reduce fertility and interfere with normal sexual behaviour. Therefore, significant increases in the rate of follicular atresia, evidence of oocyte toxicity, interference with ovulation or altered corpus luteum formation or function should be considered adverse effects.

3)   Hormone levels

Hormonal patterns and their regulation are more complex in females than in males due to the female cycle, the fertilization process, gestation and lactation. All functions of the female reproductive system are under endocrine control and therefore can be disrupted by effects on the reproductive endocrine system.

Ovarian function can be assessed hormonally in humans and experimental animals with *in vivo* and *in vitro* techniques. In animals, gonadotrophin stimulation tests are frequently used to assess steroid-ogenesis and capacity to produce ova. *In vitro* fertilization can be used to evaluate the quality of ova (fertilizability, development). In humans, data on hormone levels during fertility care can provide other supportive information.

Hormone measurements can directly indicate the function of endocrine organs. The levels of LH, FSH, prolactin, estradiol, progesterone, inhibins and testosterone reflect the rate of hormone production by the hypothalamus, pituitary and gonads. Timing of blood sampling is important, since the hormone levels depend on the estrous cycle and the age of the animal. Traditional radioimmunoassays are often too insensitive for hormone measurements in young animals or when hormone levels are suppressed; in these cases, more sensitive assays should be used, such as fluoroimmunoassays and recombinant cell assays (e.g., for estradiol, see Klein et al., 1994). Since endocrine disruption is often accompanied by structural change in endocrine target organs, morphological evaluation should also be carried out. In humans, multiple samples provide the most complete information on the cycle; however, a single sample for measurement of progesterone level approximately 7–9 days after the estimated mid-cycle surge of gonadotrophin can be sufficient to indicate normal corpus luteum, folliculogenesis and ovulation.

Hormonal levels fluctuate significantly in normal animals; thus, hormonal change is not a highly sensitive indicator of reproductive toxicity. However, greater sensitivity can be obtained if multiple measurements of hormonal levels are made; if carefully evaluated throughout the estrous cycle, significant alterations can indicate an adverse reproductive effect.

Some end-points that detect endocrine-related effects in exposed adults are part of routine testing. These include some measures of fertility, reproductive organ appearance and weight, histopathology, oocyte number, cycle patterns and mating behaviour. Uterine protein production has also been used in toxicological assessment (Maier et al., 1985). Detection of developmental effects induced by endocrine system disruption is discussed in chapter 5. Significant effects on any of these measures may be considered adverse if the results are consistent and biologically plausible.

4)   Sexual behaviour

In the rat, lordosis is a direct measure of female sexual receptivity. Sexual receptivity of the female rat is normally cyclic, with receptivity commencing during the late evening of vaginal proestrus. Agents that interfere with normal estrous cyclicity could also cause abnormal sexual behaviour that can be reflected in reduced numbers of females with vaginal plugs or vaginal sperm, alterations in lordosis behaviour and increased time to mating after start of cohabitation. However, it is not uncommon for male laboratory rats to attempt to mate with females irrespective of whether the female exhibits lordosis. In these instances, the vaginal lavage may show the presence of some sperm, but the female will not become pregnant. Since males and females are normally separated after positive evidence of mating, some care should be taken if a disproportionate number of pairings have a precoital interval of 1 day and when the pairing of males with females is not controlled with regard to female estrous.

Effects on sexual behaviour should be considered adverse. Testing of sexual behaviour is not usually available and not warranted in all cases, but should be considered for those agents that cause neurotoxicity and those that have agonistic or antagonistic adrenergic or estrogenic properties.

5)   Lactation

The mammary glands of normal adults change dramatically during the period around parturition because of the sequential effects of gonadal and extragonadal hormones. Milk letdown is dependent on the suckling stimulus and the release of oxytocin from the posterior pituitary. Thus, mammary tissue is highly dependent on hormones for development and function (Wolff, 1993; Imagawa et al., 1994; Tucker, 1994). Mammary gland size, milk production and release and histology can be affected adversely by toxic agents, and many exogenous chemicals and drugs are transferred into milk (WHO, 1988; American Academy of Pediatrics Committee on Drugs, 1994; Sonawane, 1995; LaKind et al., 2001).

6)   Reproductive senescence

Regular ovarian cycles cease in older rats, as do cyclical changes in the uterine and vaginal epithelium (Cooper & Walker, 1979). Age-dependent change in the hypothalamic–pituitary control of ovulation is the likely cause of these events (Cooper et al., 1980). In normal females, all of the follicles (and the resident oocytes) are present at or soon after birth. The large majority of these follicles undergo atresia and are not ovulated. If the population of follicles is depleted, it cannot be replaced, and the female becomes infertile. In rodents, lead, mercury, cadmium and polycyclic aromatic hydrocarbons (PAHs) have all been implicated in the arrest of follicular growth at various stages of the life cycle (Mattison & Thomford, 1989). However, different mechanisms are responsible for decreased oocyte number and decreased reproductive capacity in rodents and humans (Heindel, 1998). Environmental toxicants, estrogenic agents or antiestrogenic agents that affect gonadotrophin-mediated ovarian steroidogenesis or follicular maturation can prolong the follicular phase of the estrous or menstrual cycle and cause atresia of follicles that would otherwise ovulate. Also, normal follicular maturation is essential for normal formation and function of the corpus luteum after ovulation. These observations imply that altered ovarian function may not become evident until puberty and can influence the age at which reproductive senescence occurs. Change in the age of onset of reproductive senescence in females can be assessed using vaginal smear cytology, ovarian histopathology or an endocrine profile (see above section on the estrous cycle). Significant dose-related change in these parameters indicating altered onset of senescence should be considered an adverse effect.

.2.2   In vitro experimental data

4.2.2.1   Introduction

An extensive variety of *in vitro* test systems are available that can be used in supplementary investigational studies of the reproductive system. Examples of these systems include the maintenance of whole organs (e.g., isolated perfused testis/ovary), primary culture of gonadal cells and subcellular fractions of organs and cells. *In vitro* fertilization techniques have also started to show promise in evaluating functional end-points for toxic effects. The information obtained from such test systems can be invaluable in identifying potential mechanisms of action of xenobiotics. However, the strength of each test is usually that it simplifies the system being investigated in order to ask specific mechanistic questions; this is also a weakness, because the reproductive system is highly integrated and complex. Thus, while it may be desirable to test for reproductive toxicity with *in vitro* tests instead of with *in vivo* animal systems, this is not at present a viable alternative.

In vitro testing systems are most useful in two important areas. First, they are useful in screening for toxicity, particularly in cases where sufficient *in vivo* data exist to validate the *in vitro* results. Second, *in vitro* tests are useful to study mechanisms of toxicity, and frequently they represent the only available approach for such studies. The wide variety of *in vitro* systems available to the reproductive toxicologist has been reviewed extensively (e.g., ECETOC, 1989; Chapin & Heindel, 1993; Heindel & Chapin, 1993; OECD, 1996b; Genschow et al., 2000).

4.2.2.2 Cell and tissue culture systems

In vitro systems are particularly useful for studying the mode of action of reproductive toxicants and may provide supporting evidence for the classification of reproductive effects. The most commonly used techniques employ primary cultures of gonadal cells or cells of the reproductive tract (e.g., epididymis, uterus), including somatic (e.g., Sertoli and Leydig cells in males; granulosa, thecal and luteal cells in females) and germ cells. Co-culture of different types of gonadal cells has also been attempted to try to maintain key intercellular relationships that occur in the gonad (Tres et al., 1986). In some cases, this has been achieved by employing adjacent cell culture chambers that allow for cellular products to diffuse from one cell type to the other (Janecki & Steinberger, 1986). The effects of toxicants have also been examined in cultures of intact seminiferous tubules (Toppari et al., 1986; Allenby et al., 1991; Rodriguez & Bustos-Obregón, 2000). It is also possible to culture intact ovarian follicles (Greenwald, 1987).

4.2.2.3 In vitro fertilization studies

Many of the basic techniques for *in vitro* fertilization were established initially in the hamster (Yanagimachi et al., 1976), and the technique has been unreliable with other commonly used rodent species. A number of studies have shown that this technique can be useful to identify compounds that can interfere with fertilization or that have subtle effects on sperm (or presumably oocyte) function, which are not evident in standard evaluations of sperm number or motility. This technique has also been used in an *ex vivo/in vitro* approach (i.e., sperm or eggs from treated animals are combined with untreated gametes); alternatively, gametes can be combined and subsequently exposed to potentially toxic agents. The technique can be highly sensitive, because the number of viable sperm coming into contact with the oocyte can be carefully controlled, and results can be compared for treated and untreated gametes. Another approach uses avian reproductive tissues grafted in chicken allantois and was recently used to assess the reproductive toxicity of pesticides (Contreras et al., 1999).

Heterologous *in vitro* fertilization or, perhaps more correctly, sperm–oocyte penetration studies have also received attention. The most extensively used bioassay of this type has been the zona-free hamster oocyte test (WHO, 1999), which investigates the ability of human sperm to penetrate and fuse with the oolemma of a hamster oocyte denuded of its zona pellucida.

2.4   *Other in vitro systems*

A number of other, more specialized systems are available to the reproductive toxicologist to answer specific mechanistic questions. In particular, the hormonal control of reproductive function and its perturbation by toxicants have received much attention. Such investigations can use intact cells to investigate the downstream consequences of toxicants on hormone–receptor interactions or use cells that respond to specific hormones (e.g., the MCF-7 breast cancer cell line and estrogen; Soto et al., 1995). Receptor biology/ligand binding can be examined in membrane preparations of specific cell types or in recombinant cell systems (e.g., human and yeast cells; Klein et al., 1994) where specific hormone receptor and response elements have been transfected. This approach identifies the effects of agents on hormone–receptor interactions.

2.3   *Structure–activity relationships*

Physicochemical characteristics of a compound can be used to predict its biological activity. Computer-based molecular modelling has advanced rapidly, providing much information on structure–activity relationships. Three-dimensional quantitative structure–activity relationship (QSAR) models for ligand–receptor interactions have been developed on the basis of K_i or IC_{50} data from hormone binding assays and knowledge of steric and electrostatic properties of structurally diverse ligands (Waller & McKinney, 1995; Waller et al., 1996). At present, the QSAR models are experimental, i.e., results from QSAR analyses are compared with data from established receptor assays (Waller et al., 1996). In the future, it is hoped that QSAR will be used to predict an adverse activity of a new compound, thereby avoiding expensive biological testing. However, QSAR approaches are currently most useful to provide supporting data in conjunction with more traditional reproductive tests.

4.2.4   Methods to assess endocrine disruption

Adverse trends in reproductive health in wildlife have focused attention on the potential effects of EDCs (see Ankley et al., 1998; Campbell & Hutchinson, 1998; Crisp et al., 1998; Olsson et al., 1998; US NRC, 1999). Consequently, much effort is currently being directed towards evaluating existing international test methods and developing new methods to assess the effects of chemicals on the endocrine system (OECD, 1998a, 1998b, 1999a; US EPA, 1998d). The OECD has set up an international task force on EDCs to determine the feasibility of adding additional endocrine-related end-points to existing test guidelines and to validate the Hershberger and uterotrophic assays for known EDCs (OECD, 1999b).

4.3   Human data

4.3.1   Introduction

Well documented observational, clinical and epidemiological studies in humans provide more direct information on human health effects than do studies in animal systems. However, the number of such human data is limited, and in many cases animal data are the only information available on potential adverse reproductive effects.

4.3.2   Fecundity and fertility

Fecundity, fertility and "sperm quality" are distinct parameters that are not equivalent and are frequently confused. Sperm count and sperm quality do not necessarily predict whether conception will take place for a given couple. A "fertile couple" has conceived at least one child. Fecundity is the ability of a couple to conceive a child and is often evaluated by the time necessary to achieve pregnancy.

Infertility may be thought of as a non-event or negative outcome: a couple that is infertile is unable to have children within a specific time frame. Therefore, the epidemiological measurement of reduced fertility or fecundity is typically indirect and is accomplished by comparing birth rates or time intervals between births or pregnancies. This has been approached with several methods, including the standardized birth ratio (SBR; also referred to as the standardized fertility ratio) and the length of time to pregnancy or to birth. In these evaluations, the couple's joint ability to procreate is estimated.

The SBR compares the number of births observed with those expected based on the person-years of observation, preferably stratified by factors such as time period, age, race, marital status, parity and (if possible) contraceptive use (Baird et al., 1986; Baird, 1988). The SBR is analogous to the standardized mortality ratio, a measure frequently used in studies of occupational cohorts, and has similar limitations in interpretation (de Cock et al., 1994; Curtis et al., 1999). Welch and colleagues found that the SBR was less sensitive in identifying an effect when compared with semen analyses in the same number of men (Welch et al., 1991).

"Time to pregnancy" is also a useful tool and has clearly demonstrated a difference in fecundity among smokers and non-smokers (van der Pal-de Bruin et al., 1997). Analysis of the time between recognized pregnancies or live births is a more recent approach to indirect measurement of fertility (Wilcox, 1983; Baird & Wilcox, 1985; Baird et al., 1986; Weinberg & Gladen, 1986; Joffe et al., 1999; Apostoli et al., 2000). Because the time between births increases with increasing parity (Leridon, 1977), comparisons within birth order (parity) are more appropriate.

Because of the complexity of the reproductive system, data on age-adjusted infertility rates are sparse. The proportion of US women (age 15–44) who reported some form of fecundity impairment rose from 8% in 1982 and 1988 to 10% in 1995, an increase in absolute numbers from 4.6 to 6.2 million women (Stephen & Chandra, 1998).

In Sweden, analysis of birth registries showed that the population of subfertile women (defined as those who did not become pregnant after more than 1 year) actually decreased from 12.7% in 1983 to 8.3% in 1993 in the general population (Akre et al., 1999a). The decrease, which was independent of maternal age, was considered linked to a decrease of sexually transmitted disease incidence in Sweden.

Differences in time to pregnancy have also been found in a prospective study carried out in seven well defined geographical areas in Europe (Juul et al., 1999). The highest fecundity was in southern Italy and northern Sweden, and the lowest fecundity was in eastern Germany. The differences in time to pregnancy remained significant after adjustment for regional differences in body mass, smoking, frequency of intercourse and sexually transmitted disease. The reasons for these geographical differences have not been established. Another approach is to review the total fecundity of a population with no predisposition for limitation of family size. For example, there has been a decreased age-specific fertility rate in the Hutterite population, a group in which reproductive practices are unlikely to have changed over time (Nonaka et al., 1994; Sato et al., 1994). These retrospective cohort studies revealed a decline in the total number of children born, beginning with a cohort from 1931 to 1935 and continuing with subsequent birth cohorts. Again, the reason for this decline is unknown.

Both female and male infertility can be caused by a number of factors, e.g., impaired ovulation, impaired spermatogenesis, chromosomal abnormalities, infection and structural abnormalities of the reproductive organs. At first glance, it appears as if most clinics find a cause for infertility in about 85% of their cases. However, a closer look at the published data suggests that diagnoses such as anovulation, oligozoospermia and azoospermia are purely descriptive and are often substitutes for real knowledge of the etiology of the conditions. Fertility can also reflect alterations in sexual behaviour, but data linking exposure to these alterations in humans are limited and are not obtained easily in epidemiological studies. These data may also include information bias, which depends on the types of questions asked, the setting of the interview (telephone/doctor's office/letter; interview bias) and the memory of the interviewee (recall bias), as well as misclassification errors.

2.1   Male end-points

1)   Semen analysis

Normal gametogenesis is a prerequisite for normal fertility, although quantitatively diminished production of gametes may not prevent pregnancy. In males, spermatogenesis occurs continuously during adulthood, and the production of spermatozoa is easy to study. Semen analysis is therefore one of the basic studies of reproduction and fertility. Most epidemiological studies of semen characteristics have been conducted in occupational groups and patients receiving drug therapy. Potential parameters for study include sperm count, semen volume, morphology, motility, pH and sperm chromatin structure. Several of these use new approaches, developed over approximately the last 10 years, and will be more common in future studies.

It may be difficult to obtain a high level of participation in the workforce, because social and cultural attitudes concerning sex and reproduction influence willingness to participate in study groups. Men who are planning to have children, as well as men who are concerned about reproductive problems or possible ill effects of exposure, may be more likely to participate. Unless controlled, such biased participation can lead to misrepresentation of risk associated with exposure (US NRC, 1991; Lin et al., 1996).

In a retrospective study of 2012 farm couples, exposure to various classes of pesticides was not associated with altered time to pregnancy (Curtis et al., 1999). Similarly, a large study on exposure to pesticides in Denmark and France in which exposed individuals were compared with a control group of agricultural workers suggests that pesticide exposure has no effect on time to pregnancy (Thonneau et al., 1999). Semen of 55 male agricultural workers attending an infertility clinic in Canada had a lower average sperm concentration and an increased average number of abnormal sperm (tapered head), but the differences were not statistically significant compared with other occupational factors. More significant was a dose–response relationship found between the level of perceived job stress and various abnormalities of sperm morphology and motility (Bigelow et al., 1998). In a group of agricultural workers in Denmark, median sperm concentration was lower after the pesticide spraying season than before the season, but an equal decline was found in the control group where men were not spraying pesticides (Bonde et al., 1998a; Larsen et al., 1999).

Several factors may influence the results of semen evaluation, including the period of abstinence preceding collection of the sample, age, year of birth, season, social habits (e.g., alcohol, drugs, smoking) and health status (Jouannet et al., 1981; Auger et al., 1995; WHO, 1999). Data on these factors may be collected by interview, subject to the limitations described for pregnancy outcome studies. Semen analysis should be performed uniformly in different laboratories to gain comparable data (WHO, 1999). Computer-aided semen analysis is still in the developmental phase, but may help standardize the methodology. At present, there is little interobserver variation in the measurements of sperm concentrations, whereas assessment of motility and morphology has remained subjective in spite of the availability of detailed instructions (Jorgensen et al., 1997). Several functional tests for spermatozoa have been developed, such as sperm–cervical mucus interaction, sperm–zona pellucida interaction and the hamster egg penetration test (WHO, 1999). These can be used for limited study groups but are unlikely to be used for large population studies.

Reports of studies with semen analyses have rarely included an evaluation of endocrine status (hormone levels in blood or urine) of exposed males (Adamopoulos et al., 1996; Larsen et al., 1999). Conversely, studies that have examined endocrine status typically do not have data on semen quality (McGregor & Mason, 1990, 1991; Egeland et al., 1994). Endocrine evaluation gives important information on reproductive organs. Estradiol, progesterone, testosterone, FSH, LH and prolactin are the hormones that are most informative. Inhibins and other more recently characterized factors may provide tools in the future.

As indicated in chapter 2, much of the recent increased concern regarding human reproductive health has focused on the potential adverse effects of environmental EDCs. At the centre of this concern is the hypothesis that exposure to EDCs is associated with a decrease in sperm count/quality (Carlson et al., 1992; Sharpe, 1993; Irvine et al., 1996; Weidner et al., 1999). The available data on this hypothesis are equivocal, controversial and beyond the scope of this document (Kavlock et al., 1996; Toppari et al., 1996; Cooper & Kavlock, 1997; US NRC, 1999).

4.3.2.2   Female end-points

Numerous diagnostic methods have been developed to evaluate female reproductive dysfunction. Although these methods have rarely been used for occupational or environmental toxicological evaluations, they may be helpful in defining biological parameters and mechanisms related to female reproductive toxicity. If clinical observations link exposure to the reproductive effect of concern, these data will aid the assessment of adverse female reproductive toxicity. The following clinical observations include end-points that may be reported in case reports or epidemiological research studies.

A loss of primary oocytes will irreversibly affect a woman's fecundity, but this is difficult to measure directly. Reproductive dysfunction can be studied by the evaluation of irregularities of menstrual cycles and onset of menarche and menopause. However, menstrual cyclicity and onset of menopause and menarche are affected by many parameters, such as age, genetics, nutritional status, stress, exercise, certain drugs and the use of contraceptives that alter endocrine feedback. The length of the menstrual cycle, particularly the follicular phase (before ovulation), can vary between individuals and may make it difficult to measure significant effects in groups of women (Burch et al., 1967; Treloar et al., 1967).

One example of a new approach is the isolation of persistent organochlorine chemicals from ovarian follicular fluid of women undergoing *in vitro* fertilization (Baukloh et al., 1987; Jarrell et al., 1993; Foster et al., 2000). Isolation of such chemicals at a critical period of oocyte development can potentially provide important biomarkers of exposure and outcome. Other female end-points, including evaluation of hormone levels, fetal loss, miscarriages, etc., can also be monitored. Sensitive hCG assays help to detect pregnancies early, and therefore early embryonic loss can also be detected. Birth weight, sex ratio, congenital malformations and neonatal health can be used to measure prenatal and transgenerational effects.

Knowledge of the site and mode of action of an agent producing reproductive toxicity in animal studies can either diminish or enhance the concern for the human population. Thus, if the mode of action in the animal is via a system that is likely or known to operate in humans e.g., similar metabolic activation, action through a similar receptor system, etc. (see chapter 3), then it would tend to increase the likelihood that the agent would act through a similar mechanism and have similar effects in humans.

4.4 Summary

An enormous number of potential target sites and processes exist that could be perturbed by a toxicant and produce adverse reproductive findings. In conceptual terms, an examination of the reproductive cycle indicates many of the processes that may be targets for toxicant action. It is quite possible that one agent may have more than one potential site or mechanism of action. It should also be noted from a simple examination of the cycle that adverse effects due to exposure to a toxicant may not be immediate. Exposure *in utero* may result in latent reproductive deficits when the individual reaches adulthood and attempts to reproduce. Investigational animal studies are usually carried out to explore the mode of action of a toxicant suspected of having an adverse reproductive effect. Frequently, such potential reproductive toxicants are identified during standard regulatory testing protocols, including subacute and subchronic toxicity studies. Thus, it is reasonable to first characterize the adverse reproductive finding in terms of dose–response or pathogenesis and, if possible, link this to a functional as well as a morphological deficit. Metabolic/pharmacokinetic studies can be undertaken to analyse target tissue dosimetry, kinetics and metabolism (activation or detoxification) at relevant dose levels (i.e., those that cause adverse effects and that occur during environmental exposure). Armed with these data, specific *in vitro* (and perhaps *in vivo*) experiments can be designed to investigate biochemical perturbations in target tissues with the compound (or appropriate metabolite) at the appropriate concentration. Reasonable models should be developed and then thoroughly investigated in a sensitive animal species; finally, results should be compared in different species. *In vitro* assays could be carried out in some species that were non-responsive *in vivo* to the action of the agent. Investigation of the response of human target tissue *in vitro* may also be appropriate, when such studies are feasible.

5. EVALUATION OF DEVELOPMENTAL TOXICITY

5.1   Introduction

Developmental toxicity is taken in its widest sense to include any effect interfering with normal development both before and after birth. This subject was first brought to the attention of the public and scientific and medical professionals when it was discovered that pregnant women who took the sedative hypnotic drug thalidomide gave birth to infants with severe congenital anomalies, especially of the limbs. Prior to this discovery in 1960, thalidomide had been considered a safe alternative to other hypnotic drugs. Subsequently, worldwide testing requirements, including tests for developmental toxicity, were established for all drugs, and satisfactory test results are necessary prior to approval of a drug for distribution to the public.

The modern science of teratology essentially dates from that time. Initial guidelines placed significant emphasis on testing for safety during pregnancy, and, with thalidomide in mind, drug-induced structural anomalies were considered of primary importance. The word "teratology" is derived from the Greek "teras" meaning monster and "logos" meaning study. A "teras" (pl. terata) is a fetus with deficient, redundant, misplaced or grossly misshapen parts, and teratology is the branch of science concerned with the production, development, anatomy and classification of malformed fetuses (WHO, 1967).

It has now become clear that *in utero* exposure to drugs and chemicals can cause many different effects on the embryo or fetus in addition to gross structural anomalies (Grant, 1976; Sullivan, 1993). Nutritional factors also play an important role. The original "teratology" tests were regarded as inadequate to detect all of these effects, and the term "developmental toxicity" has been increasingly accepted in reference to the set of tests necessary to screen for these adverse effects. As part of a WHO/OECD initiative for global harmonization of risk assessment approaches, a definition for developmental toxicity has been proposed. This definition is very broad and includes any interference with development of the embryo before birth or interference with postnatal development. Thus, developmental toxicity includes adverse effects of exposure at any time during prenatal and postnatal development up to sexual maturity. Effects can manifest themselves either prenatally or postnatally; examples include reduced body weight, growth and developmental retardation, organ toxicity, death, abortion, structural (teratogenic) defects, functional defects, impaired postnatal mental or physical development, latent onset of adult disease including cancer, early reproductive senescence and shortened life span.

5.2 Background information on abnormal development

The occurrence of spontaneous anomalies is common in laboratory animals. The incidence and type of externally visible spontaneous anomalies in common laboratory strains vary over time in different laboratory animal populations, so historical control data, although extremely valuable and essential for satisfactory interpretation of studies, may also be misleading (Palmer, 1977; Szabo, 1989). Historical data from recent years provide useful background information for an experiment with a particular animal colony, but concurrent or very recent data are also necessary for data interpretation.

5.2.1 Critical periods during development

It is widely accepted that the embryo is particularly sensitive to toxic agents, and the effects tend to be irreversible. Each structure in the embryo develops at a different time and at a different rate. Empirical observations have shown that each structure is most susceptible to insults resulting in structural abnormality just prior to and during its initial formation. These organ-specific periods of extreme susceptibility have been termed critical periods or critical windows of susceptibility. Design of the prenatal developmental toxicity test recognizes the fact that the critical periods for structural development span the embryonic period; the animals are dosed throughout the embryonic period to ensure that insults that may be specific to a particular structure are detected. Originally defined as gestation days 6–15 in rats and mice and gestation days 6–18 in rabbits, this has now been extended into the fetal period in recognition that structural abnormalities of the reproductive system can be induced during that time.

As noted in chapter 3 on normal development, maturation of organ systems extends into the fetal and postnatal periods. Therefore, the notion of critical periods of susceptibility can be extended for deficits of organ function. Critical periods for functional deficit are longer than those for structural maturation and may extend postnatally (Daston & Manson, 1995; Daston, 1996b; Selevan et al., 2000).

Knowledge of critical periods may be helpful in determining the plausibility that adverse effects were produced by chemical exposure. If exposures occur only after the critical period for a structure, then abnormalities in that organ are unlikely to be attributable to the exposure. Such determinations require special study designs in which exposures are limited to only a fraction of development.

5.2.1.1 Prenatal toxicity and structural defects

It is widely accepted that the developing embryo is particularly sensitive to toxic agents during certain periods when sensitive organ systems or types of cells are at risk (Selevan et al., 2000). For example, the fetus is more sensitive to the development of structural anomalies during periods of organogenesis. However, this period cannot be defined precisely, since there is no single point at which organ development reaches completion. For practical purposes, developmental toxicity studies identify the critical period extending from implantation of the zygote to closure of the hard palate. In the rat, this critical period is defined as days 6–15 of pregnancy (day 0 is the day of mating). In the mouse and rabbit, the comparable critical periods are days 6–15 and days 6 to 18–20, respectively. The comparable period in the human is approximately days 7 to 50–60 after fertilization. A detailed timetable of comparative embryological events in laboratory and other animals is reported by Szabo (1989).

The preimplantation period is generally thought to be a period when the embryo is relatively insensitive to chemically induced malformations, although embryos can die during this period. However, the pharmacokinetics of a specific chemical during this period must be considered, because some chemicals persist in the body or in the blastocyst for several days after initial exposure. One common explanation for resistance to chemically induced anomalies early in pregnancy is that the embryo includes totipotent cells that can replace any damaged cells. However, recent evidence suggests that there is a very early window of sensitivity to chemicals. Dosing at or near fertilization with mutagens such as ethylene oxide or ethyl methane sulfonate can induce fetal malformation and death as well as reduce postnatal survival (Generoso et al., 1987, 1988; Katoh et al., 1989; Rutledge & Generoso, 1989). Katoh et al. (1989) used reciprocal zygote transfer to show that the exposure was toxic to the zygote but was not toxic to the dam. Chromosome aberrations, aneuploidy and heritable translocations were not found. Hindlimb and lower body duplications were also observed in fetuses born to mice treated with retinoic acid between postcoital days 4.5 and 5.5 (Rutledge et al., 1992; Niederreither et al., 1996).

Chemical exposure following implantation can cause a wide variety of structural abnormalities as well as death or growth retardation. The type and incidence of defects vary with the chemical, the dose and the timing of the exposure.

5.2.1.2   Fetal and postnatal developmental defects

The end of embryogenesis has been defined, for practical purposes, as the time when closure of the hard palate is complete. Although initial establishment of most organs is complete by that time, many developmental processes continue. The histological, biochemical and functional development of major organ systems, as well as brain development, proceed well into the postnatal period. In the rat, growth of the brain involving cerebellar development occurs in 2-week-old pups; in humans, brain growth and development continue during the first 2 years of life. The period when brain development is most sensitive to environmental effects extends from a few days after zygote implantation until well into the postnatal period. In the early stages, major malformations of structure, such as failure to close the neural tube, can occur; in the later stages, more subtle changes in brain biochemistry or structure can be induced. These changes can result in transient or permanent deficiencies in neurological, behavioural or intellectual functions.

5.2.2   Pharmacokinetics and pharmacodynamics

The rates of absorption, distribution, metabolism and excretion of a chemical are interrelated parameters associated with internal exposure of an organism to that chemical. These parameters determine the concentration of the compound in the maternal and fetal compartments of the organism (Mirkin & Singh, 1976). The concentration of a chemical in the body is a time-dependent value that can vary with species, route of administration, duration of exposure, physiological status of the animal and other factors. The importance of kinetic factors in developmental toxicity has only relatively recently been given the attention it deserves (Nau & Scott, 1987; Lau et al., 2000).

Chemicals ingested by a pregnant female are transferred to her fetus through the placenta. The level of fetal exposure depends on protein binding, plasma pH and degree of ionization, lipid solubility, molecular weight of the chemical, carrier systems and other factors. Chemicals also undergo metabolic transformation in the placenta, which contains phase 1 (i.e., microsomal mixed-function oxidases, mono- and diamine oxidases, aromatases, arylhydrocarbon hydroxylase) and phase 2 metabolizing enzymes (i.e., sulfatases, glucuronidases and transferases). These enzymes are important for the physiological transfer of steroid hormones and metabolites and to modify maternally derived xenobiotic chemicals. They can either decrease or increase the toxicity of xenobiotic chemicals to the developing embryo and fetus (Juchau, 1980; see review by Slikker & Miller, 1994).

Active and facilitated transport systems transport some physiologically important substances across the placenta; however, the majority of drugs and chemicals cross the placenta by simple diffusion. Because the molecules must cross a membrane structure, lipid solubility is important (Nau & Liddiard, 1978), and very lipophilic molecules such as anaesthetics are readily transported; the transfer of such molecules is limited only by the rate of placental blood flow. Nevertheless, in humans, at the maximal rate of transplacental transfer, it takes 30–60 min for equilibrium to be reached between the maternal and fetal compartments because maternal blood flow is limiting (Goldstein et al., 1968). This accounts for the clinical observation that infants born to fully anaesthetized women by caesarean section are not themselves anaesthetized. Chemicals with a molecular weight under 300 transfer rapidly; higher molecular weight chemicals cross more slowly. Special transport systems exist for transferring antibodies.

The equilibrium concentration of a chemical in the maternal and fetal circulations depends on different factors for the two circulatory systems. At equilibrium, the concentration of free diffusible chemical is the same on both sides of the placental barrier. If the chemical is bound by plasma protein and the concentration of that protein is lower in the fetus than in the mother, the concentration of the chemical will be lower on the fetal than on the maternal side. Similarly, if the chemical exists in an ionized form, then the ratio of ionized to unionized (diffusible) chemical on each side of the placenta depends on the pH in the maternal and fetal compartments. Under conditions of hypoxia or anoxia, the pH of the fetal plasma can be half a pH unit lower than that of the maternal plasma. For chemicals with a pK_a near 7, this can result in a large concentration gradient across the placenta. For lipid-soluble substances, the amount transferred to the fetus is usually low, because the body fat of the fetus is low. After birth, when the offspring starts to consume fatty food such as milk, the ability of the newborn to absorb and retain fat-soluble chemicals increases vastly (WHO, 1988).

The effects of a chemical in a tissue frequently depend on the chemical's interaction with cell surface or cytoplasmic receptors. In some cases, a chemical interacts directly with the cell membrane and alters its permeability. The pharmacodynamic actions of drugs are usually mediated by interactions with a receptor, and a drug often competes with endogenous ligands of a receptor. The toxicity of environmental chemicals can also depend on and be mediated by interactions with receptors. In some cases, the responses are different for chemical exposures at different fetal stages of development, and it is possible to explain the different responses by the chronology of the development of fetal receptor systems. The fetus may develop receptor systems for a compound before it develops the ability to metabolize that compound; thus, a low level of an active chemical can have greater and more persistent effects in the fetus than in the mother, whose metabolism limits the duration and extent of the effect. This is one mechanism for selective developmental toxicity of chemicals.

The work of Nau and his collaborators on the role of pharmaco-kinetics in teratology (Nau & Scott, 1987) has led to a clearer under-standing of the mechanism of action of some teratogens. In general, laboratory animals metabolize and excrete drugs more rapidly than humans. This observation is related to the high overall metabolic rate of small animals; small body size correlates with a high ratio of body surface area to weight and creates the need for a rapid metabolism to maintain body temperature. The level of hepatic microsomal cyto-chrome P-450 monooxygenase activity, which is involved in drug metabolism, is lower in humans than in mice, rats and hamsters (Walker, 1978; Lorenz et al., 1984). In laboratory animals, drugs tend to be absorbed well and achieve relatively high peak levels in plasma (C_{max}), but the drugs are also more rapidly distributed and excreted than in humans, leading to a shorter half-life. Using pharmacokinetics, these aspects of drug metabolism are evaluated using the area under the curve (AUC) in a plot of plasma concentration versus time, a measure of the total body exposure to the drug.

It is important to consider pharmacokinetics in teratology and ask whether C_{max} or AUC is a better indicator of exposure and the teratological potential of a chemical or drug. Studies on the antiepileptic drug valproate (Nau, 1987) show that mice dosed once daily achieve a high peak level of drug in plasma, but the AUC is low due to rapid excretion. Nau (1985) compared the teratogenic effects of valproate (induction of exencephaly) under conditions that achieve high C_{max} (single daily injection) or high AUC (slow infusion via an implanted minipump), and dose–response curves were determined for exencephaly, fetal weight retardation and embryolethality. The results showed that the dose–response curves shifted markedly to the right in animals dosed by infusion, demonstrating that for valproate, a high C_{max} has greater teratogenic impact than a high AUC.

The pharmacokinetics and pharmacodynamics of several drugs and chemicals have been studied and compared. These studies reveal that the relative importance of C_{max} and AUC differs for different drugs and can also differ for the same drug at different developmental stages. For example, cyclophosphamide and retinoids are more teratogenic in rats in small divided doses than in a larger single daily dose (Nau, 1987), indicating that AUC is more important than C_{max} in these cases. Terry et al. (1994) showed that developmental stage specificity may be as important as, or more important than, the pharmacokinetic characteristics of a particular agent. They showed that the dominant pharmacokinetic parameter is different following treatment with 2-methoxyacetic acid on day 8 or 11 of gestation in rats: C_{max} correlated with exencephaly after treatment on gestation day 8, whereas AUC correlated better with limb defects produced after treatment on gestation day 11 (Clarke et al., 1992).

If the rate of development is an important criterion for the pharmacokinetic pattern that best matches an exposure-related outcome, this becomes especially important when data are extrapolated from animals to humans, because the rate of development is much slower in humans than in most laboratory animal species. There is little information on the relative importance of C_{max} versus AUC for many environmentally relevant chemicals. This is obviously an important factor that should be considered in risk assessment. It is especially important when results are extrapolated from one species to another or when results are compared that involve different patterns of exposure. Therefore, test guidelines for the study of environmental chemicals may need to ensure adequate kinetic analysis.

5.2.3   *Gene–environment interactions*

The outcome of developmental exposures is influenced significantly by the genetics of the organism. This concept was demonstrated empirically in experimental teratology almost 50 years ago by showing that the teratogenic response to identical dosages of a corticosteroid was dependent on the strain of mouse used. Such differences occur frequently in assessments of chemicals that are conducted in multiple strains or species of laboratory animals. The basis for these differences may be in the pharmacokinetics and metabolism of the compound or may be pharmacodynamic in nature; therefore, the underlying reason for interstrain/interspecific differences may not be obvious from the reproductive toxicity study results.

Gene–environment interactions are likely to be a critically important factor accounting for the variability in human response to a toxic insult (Autrup, 2000; Bobrow & Grimbaldeston, 2000). It has been estimated that at least 25% of human structural abnormalities have a multifactorial cause; this value could actually be higher, given that the etiology for about half of all malformations is completely unknown. Studies combining molecular biology with classical epidemiological approaches have demonstrated the existence of allelic variants for developmentally important genes that may enhance the susceptibility of the embryo. For example, the association between heavy maternal cigarette smoking (>10 cigarettes/day) and cleft lip and/or palate in the offspring is marginally significant until an allelic variant for TGF-alpha is considered. The combination of smoking and the uncommon variant for the gene raises the odds ratio to a highly significant level (Hwang et al., 1995; Shaw et al., 1996).

5.2.4   Site and mechanism of action

5.2.4.1   Mechanisms of developmental toxicity

Chemicals produce adverse effects in the developing embryo and fetus by a variety of mechanisms (Bishop & Kimmel, 1997). These may involve interactions of the exogenous agent with endogenous receptors, adduction of reactive intermediates to DNA or proteins, lipid peroxidation, enzyme inhibition, cell membrane alterations and others (US NRC, 2000).

The complexity of the interactions and their outcome can be demonstrated by considering the example of retinoic acid. Retinoic acid is the active form of vitamin A. It is essential for normal development; frank vitamin A deficiency leads to abnormal development in animals. Retinoic acid is also developmentally adverse in elevated dosages in laboratory animals and humans; the 13-*cis* form of retinoic acid has been documented to produce a syndrome of craniofacial abnormalities (Webster et al., 1986) and neurobehavioural deficits (Adams & Buelke-Sam, 1981) in about 20% of the children born to women taking therapeutic levels of the retinoid periconceptionally. Retinoic acid's effects are attributable to its interactions with retinoic acid receptors in the embryo. These receptors consist of two separate types, the retinoic acid receptors and retinoid-X receptors. There are three isoforms of each; the endogenous ligand for retinoic acid receptors is all-*trans* retinoic acid, and for retinoid-X receptors is 9-*cis* retinoic acid. Upon binding ligands, these receptors dimerize; the dimers interact with specific sequences of DNA, leading directly to selective gene expression. Normal levels of retinoic acid promote gene expression that is necessary for appropriate differentiation of cells; excessive levels of retinoic acid lead to expression of genes in inappropriate locations. The consequence of this is transformation of the phenotypes of the affected cells into that of cells from a different embryonic region, leading to abnormal development. These effects are known as homeotic transformations and can be mimicked by selective overexpression or null mutation of the retinoid-responsive genes. The morphological effect is associated with changes in expression of specific pattern formation genes such as PAX-2 (Torres et al., 1995) and HOX-a10 (Mark et al., 1997). Knockout of these genes causes an identical phenotype.

5.2.4.2   *Site of action of developmental toxicants*

It is not essential for a substance to cross the placenta in order to act as a developmental toxicant. Chemicals can cause developmental toxicity by acting on the father (see section 5.3.1.3), the mother, the fetoplacental unit or the fetus directly (Bloom, 1981). In addition, postnatal development can be affected by changes in the quality or quantity of a mother's breast milk, which can occur directly or as the milk enters into the feeding pup. Chemicals may act at only one of these sites or at more than one of these sites. The role of maternal factors in developmental toxicology is discussed more fully by Daston (1994).

1)   Action on the maternal organism

The physiology of pregnancy differs quite markedly in rodents, rabbits and humans (Knobil & Neill, 1994). In humans, pituitary gonadotrophins are required after fertilization, since hCG maintains the corpus luteum. In rodents, ovarian function is required throughout gestation, and ovariectomy or removal of the corpus luteum at any stage of pregnancy results in fetal death and resorption. In humans, ovarian function is not required after approximately 1 month, since placental progesterone secretion is adequate to maintain pregnancy. These differences should be considered when extrapolating studies of teratogens from animals to humans. Chemicals that interfere with pituitary or ovarian function may be developmental toxicants in rodents at specific stages of gestation, but may not affect humans in a similar manner. In some species, interference with pituitary or ovarian hormones may result in fetal death, but congenital malformations may be seen in other species. A number of other maternal factors must also be considered carefully in evaluating developmental toxicants (see Daston, 1994).

2)   Action on the fetoplacental unit

The fetoplacental unit includes maternal and fetal placental circulations, other placental functions, umbilical cord and amniotic fluid. If chemicals — for example, vasoactive drugs — reduce the placental circulation or cause umbilical vasoconstriction, then marked prolonged action may cause fetal death from anoxia, but an action for less than 2 h in rodents may cause fetal growth retardation or malformations (Brent & Franklin, 1960; Daston, 1994). Pregnancy-induced hypertension is an important factor; unfortunately, animal models are not available.

3)   Direct action on the fetus

Chemicals that cross the placental barrier can act directly on the embryo/fetus, and it is likely that the majority of chemicals that cause developmental toxicity act in this way. Teratogenic chemicals are most likely to act directly on the fetus. Some chemicals cause maternal toxicity at high doses but interfere with embryonic or fetal development at lower doses, and these chemicals are of concern in reproductive toxicology. Many of the most widely recognized embryotoxic or teratogenic chemicals are selectively active in this manner, and the dose that causes developmental toxicity can be much lower than the dose that is toxic to the mother (Khera, 1984).

Attempts to classify chemicals according to the ratio of the dose that causes maternal toxicity to the dose that causes embryonic toxicity have been proposed for over 30 years. While the concept may seem intuitive in practice, it is very difficult to agree on exactly how this should be done. One problem is that many different toxic effects can be observed in the mother and in the embryo, so different ratios are calculated for different toxic effects; in addition, the ratios are different in different species. The subject has been reviewed by Schardein (1993).

5.2.5   Nutrition

Nutritional factors play a key role in reproductive health and may be another source of variability in reproductive toxicity study results. Laboratory animal diets are usually composed of natural products and may vary in composition depending on availability of protein and fibre sources. A great deal of attention has been paid recently to the phyto-estrogen content of stock diets, particularly those that contain high levels of soya protein. These may influence the outcome of studies in which sensitive end-points of estrogenicity are measured. However, the presence of phytoestrogens is not the sole characteristic that can influence traditional estrogenic responses; Ashby & Odum (1998) have reported that the AIN-76A diet, which is semisynthetic and contains no soya-derived protein and no phytoestrogen, increases uterine weight in sexually immature rats. Such results emphasize the need to account for variability in diet, as well as other study design features, in interpreting reproductive toxicity studies.

A more pedestrian, but important, consideration is the absolute quantity of food that is consumed in a study. Decreased food intake resulting from chemically induced toxicity may influence body weight and somatic development of offspring. It is often difficult to distinguish between such secondary effects on development and possible direct effects of a chemical on development. It is not possible to distinguish between these possibilities in standard toxicity studies unless a pair-fed control group is used.

Finally, some treatment regimens may affect the internal nutritional status of the dam, leading indirectly to abnormal development by producing a functional nutritional deficiency in the embryo. The best characterized example of this is for zinc. Toxic levels of a large number of unrelated chemical substances induce the synthesis in the maternal liver (of rodents) of metallothionein, a zinc-binding protein. While this may have survival advantages for the mother, it leads to a transitory decrease in circulating zinc concentration and a functional zinc deficiency in the embryo, which may be developmentally adverse (Keen et al., 1989; Daston, 1994; Rogers et al., 1995; Jankowski-Hennig et al., 2000).

5.3 Experimental data

5.3.1 *In vivo experimental data: structural and functional aspects*

5.3.1.1 *Prenatal observations*

Prenatal observations should include examination of both pregnant animals and their embryos/fetuses. Dams should be examined regularly for signs of toxicity. Body weight should be measured and food and water intake monitored; changes in these parameters are useful indicators of toxicity, and intake must be measured carefully if chemicals are administered in the food or water. The length of gestation should be recorded. Known pharmacological or toxic effects of a chemical under study, such as sedation, respiratory depression or haemolysis, should be monitored during treatment, and the possibility that other observed effects are secondary to the toxic responses should be considered. These observations should be used to assess the maternal toxicity and determine if it contributes to embryo/fetal toxicity. Biomarkers of organ toxicity could be employed to a greater extent to monitor toxicity.

The uterus and its contents should also be examined prior to parturition to determine the number of live young and dead embryos and fetuses. The sum of these values equals the number of implantation sites. If the corpora lutea are counted (this may be very difficult in mice), then the difference between the number of implants and the number of corpora lutea indicates the extent of preimplantation loss. However, this is not necessarily accurate if the dam is dosed at the time of implantation, because it is possible to interfere with implantation to the extent that no visible sign remains. The difference between the total number of implants and the number of live implants gives the post-implantation loss, subject to the same caution as above. If there are no signs of implantation, the uterus can be stained with ammonium sulfide (Saleweski, 1964), which reveals completely resorbed implantation sites. The difficulty of distinguishing between preimplantation loss and very early postnatal implantation loss emphasizes the necessity of evaluating both parameters.

Viable fetuses should be labelled for identification, examined for visible malformations, visceral and skeletal anomalies and variations, sexed and weighed. Since there is an inverse correlation between number of fetuses per litter and individual fetal weight, total litter weight is also a useful measurement.

It is helpful to distinguish between early and late embryonic deaths (resorptions), because dose-related effects can assist in determining the greatest period of sensitivity to an agent being tested. The weight of the placenta and its physical characteristics may also be of value in interpreting results (see OECD, 2001b). In studies of rats, mice and hamsters, it is common to alternately allocate fetuses for visceral or skeletal examination, so that half of each litter is examined for each type of defect. When fetal sectioning (Wilson, 1965) is used for visceral examination, then the fetus cannot be examined skeletally. When microdissection is used, then the fetuses can be examined both viscerally and skeletally. For rabbits or other larger fetuses, every fetus should be examined for both visceral and skeletal effects. A variety of techniques are available for skeletal examination, including single staining with alizarin (Dawson, 1926), double staining with alizarin and alcian blue, which shows both ossified bone and cartilage (Inouye, 1976; Whitaker & Dix, 1979), and X-rays with or without intensification (Nothdurft & Sterz, 1977). The experience and training of the scientific personnel performing these analyses and quality of the available facilities are important considerations in deciding which techniques to use, because these factors can influence the quality of the experimental results.

There is no agreement on which statistical methods should be used for evaluating experimental data on developmental toxicity. However, some of the factors relevant to this issue are discussed in the US EPA (1991) and OECD (2001a, 2001b) guidelines. Group mean (± standard deviation) should be reported for fetuses and litters, and values for individual fetuses and individual litters should also be reported. Malformations, anomalies and variations should be reported with clear indication of the individual fetuses and litters involved, as well as the precise number of affected fetuses and their distribution in litters. This information is essential so that the data can be independently analysed by another investigator. Results should be analysed for dose–response, specificity and frequency, and treated animals should be compared with vehicle or with untreated control animals.

5.3.1.2 Postnatal manifestations

As discussed above, organ systems and the entire organism mature slowly over a long period that extends well into the postnatal period and up to puberty. Thus, organisms are at risk for exposure-induced functional defects for a longer period than they are at risk for structural malformation. Functional abnormalities have been linked to exposure during the prenatal or early postnatal period. However, functional abnormalities can be difficult to detect, and it may be necessary to use specially designed functional or behavioural tests for such changes. Pre- and postnatal chemical exposure can affect neurological function, simple and complex behaviour, reproduction, endocrine function, immune competence, xenobiotic metabolism and the function of hepatic, renal, respiratory and cardiovascular organ systems. A recent workshop evaluated critical periods of vulnerability for various organ systems in the developing organism (Selevan et al., 2000).

It is beyond the scope of this monograph to discuss all these subjects; however, the interested reader is referred to major textbooks on developmental (Kimmel & Buelke-Sam, 1994) and general toxicology (Klaassen et al., 1996) and previous IPCS monographs (IPCS, 1984, 1986a, 1986b). The methods used to assess the function of these systems in prenatally exposed progeny are similar to those conventionally used in toxicology. Specific methods that have been developed to assess physical, neurological and behavioural development are discussed in more detail below. Methods for the study of reproductive function were discussed in chapter 4.

1)   Methods for assessing behaviour

The term "behavioural teratology" was first used by Werboff & Gottlieb (1963), who studied rats exposed prenatally to tranquillizer drugs. They described the effects of these drugs in treated rats as interference with "the behavioural or functional adaptation of the offspring to its environment." The term behavioural teratology has since been used to describe postnatal deficits induced by prenatal exposure to chemicals (Barlow & Sullivan, 1975). As discussed below, there is now a wider focus on broadly defined developmental toxicology and neurotoxicology, including structural and functional effects detected both pre- and postnatally. Permanent functional deficits may be caused by macro- or microstructural defects or by changes in neurochemical and neurotransmitter synthesis, storage and release or receptor function. Behavioural changes may precede neuropathological changes and provide a more sensitive indication of a chemical's toxicity (Spyker, 1975; Weiss, 1975; Tilson & Mitchell, 1980; IPCS, 1986b; Kimmel & Gaylor, 1988; Tilson, 1990, 1998; Landrigan et al., 2000).

Exposure to chemicals during development can result in a plethora of effects, ranging from gross structural abnormalities and altered growth to more subtle effects (Spyker, 1975). The qualitative measures of some injuries during development may differ from those seen in the adult, such as changes in tissue volume, misplaced or misoriented neurons, altered connectivity or delays/acceleration of the appearance of functional or structural end-points (Rodier, 1986). In some cases, the results of early injuries become evident only as the nervous system matures and ages (Vorhees, 1986; Rodier, 1990; Harry, 1994; Kimmel & Buelke-Sam, 1994). The specificity of the damage may be a function of the timing of cell proliferation or differentiation at the time when effects are expressed.

2)   Methods of assessing development and function

Regulatory acceptance of behavioural tests to assess function became evident when behavioural end-points were included in OECD and US EPA toxicity test guidelines. These tests have been reviewed extensively, and a number of them have been standardized and validated (Buelke-Sam et al., 1985; Kimmel et al., 1990; Tilson et al., 1997). The different classes of tests to assess function are briefly summarized below:

■ *Physical development*: Growth and survival are important indicators of normal function. From the point of view of screening, body weight gain and deviations from a normal range of body weight at a given time in development may be significant indications of developmental toxicity (Adams & Buelke-Sam, 1981). Most physical landmarks correlate so well with body weight that it may be unnecessary to record the timing of physical landmarks such as pinna detachment, hair growth, incisor eruption and ear and eye opening (Hughes & Palmer, 1980).

■ *Reflex development*: The timing of acquisition of different reflexes is frequently measured (Smart & Dobbing, 1971). These include static and dynamic righting reflexes, negative geotaxic response, auditory startle reflex and grasping and placing reflexes. It is important to ensure not only that all pups acquire the reflexes but that they do so within a reasonable range of time, which has to be determined for the individual species, strain and housing and nutritional conditions, which all influence the rate of development of reflexes.

■ *Sensory development*: Several screening tests that detect overall sensory deficits rely on orientation or the response of an animal to a stimulus. Responses are recorded as present, absent or changed in magnitude (Moser & MacPhail, 1989). Another approach to the characterization of sensory function involves the use of reflex modification techniques (Crofton, 1990). Changes in stimulus frequency or threshold required to elicit a reflex or to induce habituation indicate possible changes in sensory function.

■ *Motor functions*: The timing of the normal development of motor functions has been described by Alder & Zbinden (1977). Spontaneous activity can be assessed in a familiar home cage environment and also in the more unfamiliar open field, which is also used to provide much more than just locomotor information. Spontaneous activity can be assessed for short periods or over longer periods by automatic activity-measuring equipment. This approach can provide an integrated assessment of activity during the night when rodents are most active. Specific aspects of motor and sensorimotor coordination performance are studied by elicited motor activity tests, such as crossing a narrow path, climbing a rope or balancing on a rotating rod. Analysis of swimming movements has also been useful. Standard neurobehavioural methods are available for such tests (Holson et al., 1990; ECETOC, 1992; IPCS, 2001a).

■ *Cognitive development*: Cognitive development is essentially defined as the ability to learn or respond appropriately to environmental change. Numerous methods are available for evaluating cognitive function in laboratory animals. Many reviews of these methods have been published, along with examples of chemicals that affect cognitive development (IPCS, 1986a, 1986b; ECETOC, 1992; Tilson et al., 1997; US NRC 2000).

3.1.3 Male-mediated developmental toxicity and transplacental carcinogenesis

Preconceptual and transplacental carcinogenesis are special types of developmental toxicity and can result when either parent is exposed prior to mating. Both male-mediated and female-mediated effects have been demonstrated in experimental animals for a variety of chemicals and several types of radiation (Anderson, 2000). Transplacental carcinogenesis is recognized in the female, but carcinogenesis mediated through the male germ cells is not as well appreciated or understood.

Congenital anomalies and tumours can be studied in the offspring of exposed male rodents mated to untreated females. The pups are examined the day before term, as opposed to mid-term, as in the conventional study (Knudsen et al., 1977). At this stage, congenital anomalies can be detected and documented, including hydrocephaly, exencephaly, cleft palate, open eye, runts (dwarfs), oedema, anasarca and gastrochisis. Some of these abnormalities are similar to those that occur in humans. The fetuses can also be examined for skeletal malformations by using alizarin staining. If the treated and control parental males are mated with more than one female, then some pups fathered by the same male can also be examined as liveborn offspring for the same abnormalities. Litters can also be allowed to develop to adulthood and tumour incidence monitored (Anderson et al., 1996, 1998).

Many factors influence the outcomes of these studies, including the exact time of mating, species/strain used and local husbandry conditions. It is important to obtain sufficient numbers of offspring for analysis in these studies; thus, the number of deaths caused by lethal mutation should be optimized to allow detection of both lethal and non-lethal effects. As with any toxicological model, careful control of parameters is required. However, this assay system is a useful model to examine inherited congenital malformations and tumours in the progeny of exposed males, and this kind of data could be useful for predicting effects in humans.

Studies on maternally mediated transplacental carcinogenesis have been conducted for a few chemicals, including nitroso compounds, PAHs, aminoazo compounds and mycotoxins. While almost all sites may be affected in the fetus, the most common sites are the nervous system, kidney, lung and reproductive system (Alexandrov, 1976; Rice, 1981; Diwan et al., 1999; Rice & Wilbourn, 2000). The most sensitive fetal period is late pregnancy, when the enzymes to metabolize carcinogenic chemicals develop in the fetus. Frequently, the doses required to produce tumours in the fetus are lower than those required to produce tumours in the adult. For example, a rat fetus may be 20–50 times more sensitive to the carcinogenic action of nitrosoethylurea than an adult rat (Ivankovic & Druckrey, 1968; Donovan, 1999); the opposite is occasionally true as well (e.g., the rat fetus is 10 times less sensitive to nitrosodimethylamine than the adult rat; Alexandrov, 1976). The latent period before a tumour appears can be much shorter in the fetus than in the adult. In some cases (e.g., DES), there is evidence that increased susceptibility to cancer persists for several generations following transplacental exposure (Nomura, 1982; Newbold et al., 1998, 2000).

Tests for transplacental carcinogenicity are similar to tests for carcinogenicity in an adult animal (IARC, 1980; Neubert, 1980; OECD,

1981b). Studies are normally carried out in mice or rats; rats tend to show more variability in fetal:adult sensitivity than mice. Strains of mice with specific cancer susceptibilities may be of particular value; it is also expected that studies using transgenic and knockout animals will be very informative (Nebert et al., 2000). For rodents, treatment during the last 10 days of pregnancy gives optimum sensitivity; successful studies were reported using multiple doses or using single-day dosing (Alexandrov, 1976). If treatment is given close to parturition, then it is important to avoid exposure of the feeding pup to the chemical via breast milk, and cross-fostering of offspring may be necessary. Follow-up may be required for the full life span of the offspring; however, in most cases, tumours often appear in relatively young animals.

5.3.2   In vitro systems

A number of *in vitro* developmental systems have been used to investigate the morphological and biochemical basis of normal and abnormal development. Examples include cell, organ and whole embryo culture. Although it is unlikely that *in vitro* systems will ever be able to replace whole animal systems for risk assessment, *in vitro* tests are very useful when used in addition to *in vivo* studies (Stahlmann et al., 1993). In particular, they are useful to study the mechanisms of normal and abnormal development, to determine dose–response, to identify organ toxicity and perhaps to screen or prioritize chemicals for further *in vivo* studies. However, most *in vitro* tests focus on a narrow range of developmental events; thus, some researchers feel that *in vitro* studies should be based on previously characterized results from *in vivo* studies (Schwetz, 1993).

A wide range of *in vitro* systems are available for the study of reproductive and developmental toxicity, and these have been reviewed extensively (Brown & Fabro, 1981; ECETOC, 1989; Kimmel & Kochhar, 1990; Welsch, 1990; Brown, 1994; Daston, 1996a). Current *in vitro* systems include whole embryo culture, organ and tissue culture and non-mammalian systems. Some systems have been developed for detailed investigation of normal development, including studies of anatomy/morphology and molecular biology. There is a need for systems that can be used to screen large numbers of chemicals rapidly and inexpensively for teratogenic activity. Some success along these lines has been claimed for related and homologous series of compounds (Wolpert & Brown, 1995).

5.3.2.1   Embryonic stem cell test

The embryonic stem cell test is an *in vitro* embryotoxicity test that uses permanent mouse cell lines that can differentiate into a variety of distinct cell types *in vitro* (Spielmann et al., 1997). The test has been validated in different laboratories utilizing known test chemicals with different embryotoxic properties (Scholz et al., 1999; Genschow et al., 2000). Chemicals are assigned to one of three classes of embryo-toxicity: negative, moderate and strong.

5.3.2.2   Whole embryo culture

1)   Rat

The most successful methods for whole rat embryo culture are based on work by New and colleagues (e.g., New, 1978). This method involves explantation of 9.5-day rat embryos into culture bottles containing heat-inactivated male rat serum gassed with an oxygen/carbon dioxide mixture. The embryos are incubated for 24 or 48 h at 37 °C, and the morphology, somite number, crown–rump length and head length are assessed using standardized criteria (Brown & Fabro, 1981).

Because of its obvious attractions, this system has been widely used in academic and industrial research laboratories. Interlaboratory comparisons have shown that under standardized conditions, consistent results can be obtained using known teratogens and non-teratogens. Considerable expertise is required, however, to distinguish between specific and non-specific effects and to interpret different types of embryotoxicity (Piersma et al., 1995). Although differences in rat strains may be relatively unimportant in detecting toxic effects (Piersma et al., 1995), control incidences of abnormalities do vary in different rat strains, so conditions have to be optimized prior to testing (Bechter & Terlouw, 1993).

The range of developmental stages that can be cultured is limited, usually from the 0–8 somite stage at the start of culture to the 20–22 stage after 24 h, and there is some evidence that early somite stages may be slightly more sensitive to chemical toxicity than later somite stages (Piersma et al., 1991). Variations in the culture technique, such as growth in human serum from normal or diseased individuals, have been used with varying degrees of success (Van Maele-Fabry et al., 1991). Additions have also been made to the system, including microsomal metabolizing systems with cofactors (Fantel et al., 1979; Kitchin et al., 1981) or hepatocytes (Oglesby et al., 1986; Piersma et al., 1991).

A combined *in vivo*/*in vitro* system for chemical metabolites has been developed that demonstrates the role of metabolism in activating compounds. In this system, rats are treated with a chemical and serum is removed 1 h later and cultured with explanted embryos. This system has been used to demonstrate that metabolites of procarbazine are toxic to explanted embryos, but that procarbazine and a microsomal preparation are not toxic to explanted embryos grown in culture medium (Schmid et al., 1982).

The yolk sac is present in the culture system, and it may influence the experimental results. For example, some teratogens, such as trypan blue, are specific for species that have yolk sacs (Gillman et al., 1948; Beck & Lloyd, 1963). Other advantages and disadvantages of the rat embryo culture system have been recently reviewed by Schmid et al. (1993).

2)   Other mammalian species

Mouse embryos have been cultured using a system similar to the rat whole embryo culture system. Mouse embryos and rat embryos are cultured during similar developmental stages, but mouse embryos grow slightly more slowly than rat embryos (Van Maele-Fabry et al., 1991). The mouse system has been less extensively used for chemical toxicity screening. Both the mouse and rabbit have been successfully used to investigate the effects of chemicals on the early preimplantation stage of development, for studying normal development (Mummery et al., 1993) and for chemical testing (Alm et al., 1996; Lindenau & Fischer, 1996).

3)   Chicken embryo

Although the hen egg has been a tool in embryology for decades, it has generally been agreed that it is too sensitive and non-specific to be of value in chemical toxicity screening, although some workers have used it extensively with good success (Jelinek & Peterka, 1981). In a recent modification of the system, the embryo is removed from the egg after 20 h of incubation, explanted onto defined salt solution with added egg albumin and cultured for 3 days. This modified protocol has proved very useful and reliable and gives results that correlate well with the rat embryo culture system (Schmid et al., 1993).

Efforts have been made to validate the use of whole chicken embryo cultures for chemical toxicity investigations, and these studies have been reviewed by Schmid and colleagues (Schmid et al., 1993). The results show that reproducible and predictive results can be obtained and that this approach, when supplemented by other test systems, can improve the reliability of the predictions of chemical toxicity.

4)   Other non-mammalian systems

A few non-mammalian whole embryo culture systems using fish, amphibia and invertebrates have been proposed for developmental toxicity testing. Their usefulness has been very limited, although they may have some value for screening and prioritizing chemicals for further testing (Christian, 1993). Two tests that have been more widely used than the others are the hydra developmental toxicity assay (Johnson et al., 1988) and the FETAX (*Xenopus*) assay (Dawson & Bantle, 1987; Dawson, 1991). Neither of these test systems has been generally accepted as useful for predicting human hazards, although the FETAX test may have value for studying effects in ecosystems.

5.3.2.3   Organ culture systems

The term organ culture is used when a whole organ anlage or a representative part, such as a lung lobe, is grown in culture and organ-specific differentiation is observed. Both surface and submerged growth conditions have been used (Neubert, 1982). Organ culture systems include pancreas, palatal shelves, tooth anlage, eye lens, kidney, gonads, bone, lung, intestine and liver (reviewed in IPCS, 1984). Limb bud culture has been extensively studied in a variety of species, including rat, mouse, rabbit, chick and ferret. A review of the effects of antiviral drugs on limb bud and fetal thymus cultures has been published (Stahlmann et al., 1993).

3.2.4   Cell and tissue culture

Tissue culture has been used to a limited extent for developmental toxicity studies; of the studies that have used tissue culture systems, those using chick neural crest cells (Greenberg, 1982) and human embryonic palatal mesenchyme (Pratt et al., 1980, 1982) have been especially useful. In addition, the "micromass" teratogen test, first described by Flint & Orton (1984), has been used as a screening tool, and this test has been used successfully for many years. This method uses cultures of limb and CNS cells. Rat cells are normally used, but mouse and chick cells have also been studied. Many different end-points can be assessed. For a detailed description of the method, the validation studies and discussion of its predictive value, see Flint (1993). Chick embryo neural retina cells have also been grown in culture (Daston et al., 1995), and studies indicate positive responses to chemicals at concentrations similar to those active in *in vivo* tests. Reinhardt (1993) has reviewed the use of organ slices, aggregate cell cultures and the micromass techniques for the study of neurodev-elopmental toxicity. Two recent reviews of these *in vitro* systems, especially the micromass and the chick embryo neural retinal cell system, have been published (Daston, 1996a; Mirkes, 1996).

5.3.3   Human developmental toxicity studies

Assessing developmental toxicity in humans requires a sample of individuals, information about their exposure, measurement of the out-come that might by altered by the toxicant and knowledge of the sample characteristics that might affect any observed relationship between the exposure and outcome. An overview of the methods used in human studies of this type is found in chapter 6. In this section, we outline the outcomes that are used most frequently to study develop-mental toxicity. Some may reflect events during the pregnancy and are measurable immediately after it ends. Other outcomes that arise from pregnancy or postnatal events cannot be observed until later, perhaps until adulthood. We also touch on issues that are relevant to exposure and give examples of agents that are developmental toxicants in humans.

5.3.3.1   Outcomes measured in the newborn period

In experimental animals, the outcomes used to evaluate developmental toxicity at the end of pregnancy are total implantations (with number of live young and early and late fetal losses specified), sex and weight of viable progeny, as well as malformations and anomalies. Some of these are comparable to the most useful pregnancy outcomes for evaluating developmental toxicity in humans. Specifically, in humans, one can measure pregnancy loss (embryo/fetal death at any point before or during parturition), congenital malformations that are readily identified in the newborn, gestational length and the weight of the infant at birth and, for groups of infants, the sex ratio (number of males/number of females × 100).

As in animals, early and late fetal losses should be separated. For studies that cover less than 20 weeks of human gestation, survival is probably the only usable end-point. However, it is useful only to the extent that the losses can be reliably identified. Losses in the first half of pregnancy are often not known or recorded, so survival rates are difficult to determine. Improved methods for identifying embryonic loss have been developed, and sensitive urinary hCG assays can be used (Wilcox et al., 1985; Zinaman et al., 1996), but they are demanding for both research subject and investigator. Clinical records are not useful, because many early losses are either not recognized or not reported. The later the gestational cut-off, the more likely that deaths will be reported accurately, but the rarer they will be. After 20 weeks, the rate of survival is more reliably determined, either from individual records or from vital statistics on fetal death. However, even within an area as homogeneous as Europe, late fetal deaths are not uniformly defined across countries, nor are the criteria for entry into vital statistics registries necessarily comparable (Gourbin & Masuy-Strobant, 1995).

After 20 weeks, growth *in utero* is a very useful measure of developmental toxicity, because it predicts survival better than any other characteristic (Wilcox et al., 1999). (In many countries, this is reported for liveborn infants only.) Growth has three facets: length of gestation, weight at birth and weight for gestational length (intrauterine growth). Gestational length is imprecise unless ultrasound measurements, especially for the first half of pregnancy, are available (Mul et al., 1996). Weight can be measured more accurately; if it is below

2500 g, it is defined as "low birth weight." Low birth weight is generally regarded as an adverse outcome, although this does not take into consideration the many factors, such as sex of infant, ethnic characteristics and altitude of residence, that could modify this conclusion. Weight for gestational length is more meaningful and permits one to distinguish between babies born too early and babies who failed to grow normally *in utero*, regardless of the length of the pregnancy. These adverse growth patterns may have different etiologies (Kramer, 1987; Moore et al., 1994).

Congenital anomalies that are reliably identified at birth are relatively rare in humans, but such structural malformations have been identified in about 2–3% of liveborn babies across almost all countries that collect such data (International Clearing House, 1991). If one includes progeny that do not survive, the rate is considerably higher. Such anomalies can be due to a toxic prenatal exposure (e.g., thalidomide) or to an inherited disorder (Wilkie et al., 1994). They could also reflect developmental toxicity, depending on the timing of the exposure and the critical window for the type of malformation. An accurate assessment of the prevalence of birth defects in a sample or a population requires rigorous examination of every infant, using a standardized protocol. This is seldom done for birth defect registries, so it is not surprising that they have not been useful in identifying new teratogens that have limited effects (Khoury & Holtzman, 1987).

The sex ratio has been used to monitor developmental toxicity. Declining sex ratios (fewer males) have been recorded over the last 50 years for a number of regions, including Denmark, the Netherlands, Canada and the USA (Allan et al., 1997; Safe, 2000). Several reports have implicated pesticide exposure, but the change in rate of male births in Finland in the last 250 years antedated any increase in exposure to environmental chemicals (Vartianen et al., 1999). The problem is difficult to study, because a very large population is required to determine if any changes observed are random variations or reflections of toxicant exposure.

Large samples are also required for most studies of infrequent outcomes, such as stillbirth, specific congenital malformations and low birth weight; small samples may lack the power to reveal a true association between the exposure and adverse event, if one exists. Registries can alleviate the problem if they are complete and well maintained. For example, if all infants are examined and every case of a given malformation is identified and registered, with accurate supplemental data, these cases can be compared with infants without the malformation. Omission of numerous cases is problematic because they may differ from the registry cases in some systematic way that alters any conclusion based on the registry data. Studies of the more common outcomes, such as birth weight (expressed as a continuous variable), do not require such large samples and may be preferred for that reason. Combining different outcomes (such as several types of congenital malformations) to increase sample size may be risky because they may have different etiologies and thus may be differentially sensitive to toxicant exposure.

Which pregnancy outcomes are most useful to describe developmental toxicity? This question has been addressed by Savitz and co-workers (Savitz & Harlow, 1991; Savitz, 1994; Savitz et al., 1997), who note that multiple outcomes should be measured, since essentially every facet of reproduction and development could be affected by an exogenous agent. In theory, the more end-points are measured, the greater the likelihood of detecting a toxicant effect and its mechanism of action. In fact, the choice of end-points may be limited by practical constraints, such as the number of pregnancies available for study, the type of information gathering required and the resources at the investigator's disposal.

5.3.3.2   *Outcomes measured in infancy and childhood*

Humans mature slowly, so they are at risk for functional defects for an extended period after birth. Outcomes observed in humans include changes in growth, behaviour and organ or system function and development. Cognitive, neurological, motor and sensory evaluations are used, and reproductive function is evaluated. All of these are vulnerable to the effects of toxicants. Childhood cancer is a specific end-point that is rare but possible. The critical exposure window for an adverse outcome will vary depending on the chemical exposure (Rogan et al., 1986; Jacobson & Jacobson, 1996). There is limited evidence in humans that exposure of one of the parents prior to conception of the progeny could also result in an adverse outcome (Aschengrau & Monson, 1989; Jarrell et al., 1996).

The lack of data on environmental exposure and postnatal effects reflects the enormous complexity of documenting such changes in children. Methods in developmental toxicity assessment must reflect this diversity of postnatal functions. The studies are expensive because they are generally prospective and longitudinal; that is, a group is recruited and then followed over time to observe its development. Jacobson & Jacobson (1996) have reviewed methodological issues associated with the design of prospective, longitudinal developmental studies. Standardized developmental scales must be adapted for specific countries and cultures. The selection of appropriate testing methods and conditions is very important when assessing children because of shorter attention spans and increased dependence on parental and environmental supports. The end-points frequently used to assess developmental neurotoxicity in exposed children have been reviewed by Winneke (1995); this is an important area, because the brain is very vulnerable to insult over a long period of time (Weiss, 2000; IPCS, 2001a). In addition, because of the increasing complexity of functional capabilities during early development, only a few tests appropriate for infants can be readminstered to older children.

Exposure patterns as well as developmental characteristics change as the child matures, and this must be taken into account. Both biological and behavioural changes affect the potential for exposure (reviewed in Cohen-Hubal et al., 2000). For example, small children mouth toys that may contain harmful chemicals. Children's diets are different, including liquid intake. Because of differences in metabolism, they may reach higher levels with a given exposure than those for adults. This combination of exposure and outcome complexities makes assessment of childhood developmental toxicity an extremely difficult endeavour.

5.3.3.3 *Outcomes measured in adulthood*

In the last decade, a number of reports have been published describing adverse organ or system function in adulthood that could be ascribed to prenatal insult. One example is the appearance of cancer among young women whose mothers took DES during the pregnancy (Herbst et al., 1971). A growing number of investigations also link adult blood pressure and several chronic diseases to disturbed intra-uterine growth (Cheung et al., 2000). These examples underscore the possibility of latent effects of developmental toxicity, and studies to explore this area should be undertaken.

5.3.4 *Special considerations for developmental toxicity studies in humans*

An important complication that is specific to human developmental toxicity studies is the necessity to control for confounding factors that influence human development, such as parental intelligence, quality of home environment, nutritional factors and socio-economic status (Bellinger et al., 1992; Bellinger, 1995). These may influence the outcomes from the newborn period to adulthood. In addition, assessment methods must take into consideration the time (days, months or years) that may intervene between exposure/insult and the expression of toxicity at a much later age.

It is important to assess multiple outcomes, since a variety of effects may be correlated if a toxicant has multiple targets or if it has a latent effect. For example, intrauterine growth retardation is a well established correlate for many male reproductive problems, such as testicular cancer (Moller & Skakkebaek, 1997), cryptorchidism and hypospadias (Akre et al., 1999b). The correlation of outcomes is a reflection of the intricate biological interactions of the human organism.

The human reproductive process does not fit perfectly into the animal model of reproductive and developmental toxicity. Conditions of the fetal–maternal unit that affect both mother and child have not been adequately addressed in this monograph, although there is some evidence that some of these adverse outcomes, such as pregnancy-induced hypertension, may be related to environmental exposure (Tabacova et al., 1998; Dawson et al., 1999). This is a promising frontier for new research. We have also not dealt with genetic susceptibility to developmental toxicants. Advances in this field may illuminate many of the mysteries of how toxicants act, and on whom. Limited data are available on mechanisms of action (see section 5.2.4). The work on oxidative stress in pregnancy (Tabacova et al., 1998; Hubel, 1999) is an example of how toxicants may act to affect development.

Regardless of the type of human study, ethical considerations are of paramount importance and may vary in different countries.

Guidelines for the conduct of clinical trials of pharmaceutical agents have been published (e.g., WHO, 1995), and internationally recognized EC Principles of Good Clinical Practice have been developed (EC, 1990). However, international Good Epidemiology Practice guidelines have not yet been published. In all cases where scientific research involves human participants, internationally accepted ethical codes should be taken into consideration.

5.4   Summary

Although our understanding of the potential subtle and long-lasting developmental effects of reproductive toxicants has advanced significantly during the last decade, the information on the extent to which exposures to environmental chemicals result in neurodevelopmental changes remains limited. Most developmental disabilities in children remain of unknown etiology. Although the magnitude of the effects may be small, they may have significant impact on public health. Comprehensive, prospective, longitudinal studies on the effects of exposure to chemicals on child development are needed.

6. RISK ASSESSMENT STRATEGIES FOR REPRODUCTIVE TOXICITY

6.1 Introduction

Risk assessment is an empirically based process that estimates the risk of adverse effects from exposure of an individual or population to a chemical, physical or biological agent. The OECD test guidelines, the US EPA risk assessment guidelines and additional risk assessment procedures for new and existing chemicals have been published and put into use by many different countries in Europe, the Americas and Asia (United Kingdom Department of Health, 1991, 1995; EC, 1994, 1996; Health Canada, 1994; IPCS, 1994; Hertel, 1996). A list of assessments produced by various national and international agencies on specific chemicals is included in ECETOC/UNEP (1996).

Risk is defined as the probability of adverse effects in an organism, a population or an ecological system caused under specified conditions by a chemical, physical or biological agent (OECD/IPCS, 2001). The risk assessment process usually involves four steps: hazard identification, dose–response assessment, exposure assessment and risk characterization (US NRC, 1983; WHO, 1999). The first two components of the risk assessment process, hazard identification and dose–response assessment, constitute the basic toxicological evaluation. This evaluation is aimed at characterizing the sufficiency and strength of the available toxicity data and may indicate some level of confidence in the data. Each source of information has its advantages and limitations, which determine the "weight of the evidence." Dose–response modelling may be included, if data are available. The third component, exposure assessment, estimates potential human exposure based on various environmental and/or occupational scenarios. The integration of human exposure and animal testing data with exposure assessment is termed risk characterization and constitutes the final step in the risk assessment process (Kimmel et al., 1986).

Risk management is the process that applies information obtained through the risk assessment process to determine whether the assessed risk should be reduced and, if so, to what extent. In some cases, risk is the only factor considered in a decision to regulate exposure to a substance. Alternatively, the risk posed by a substance is weighed against social, ethical and medical benefits and economic and techno- logical factors in weighing alternative regulatory options and making regulatory and public health decisions. Risk management is purposely separated from the scientific evaluation (i.e., risk assessment) for the following reason: the scientific data should be fully evaluated in a con- text free from the influence of non-scientific issues and pressures. Relevant social, economic, political, public health or other issues should be considered independently. The risk-balancing approach is used by some agencies to consider the benefits as well as the risks associated with use of the chemical. Additional sources of information on reproductive toxicity risk assessment include IPCS (1984, 1986a), ECETOC (1989), Moore et al. (1995), EC (1996) and Moore (1997).

Regulatory agencies around the world have set standards over the last three decades for limiting exposure to hazardous agents and preventing reproductive toxicity. The regulations issued by these agencies are based largely on experimental data on reproductive toxic- ity. The approaches to assess the risk to reproductive health include testing protocols in animals exposed to chemicals during critical win- dows of the reproductive cycle. As described previously, tests were initially designed to detect chemically induced structural anomalies, but more recent strategies have been developed to evaluate risk of func- tional deficiencies as well as structural anomalies.

This chapter describes current strategies and approaches to assess- ing developmental and reproductive toxicity and identifies research needs to improve the scientific basis for risk assessment. It is intended to provide the reader with an appreciation of the complexity of repro- ductive toxicity risk assessment.

6.2 Testing strategies and protocols

Strategies and protocols for detecting reproductive toxicity differ for different substances. Background information relevant to the proposed tests and the purpose of the tests can also influence the strategy or protocol used. Acceptable protocols also differ in different geographic locations with different regulatory authorities. OECD test- ing guidelines for chemicals were developed and adopted by interna- tional agreement, and this has greatly advanced the international acceptance of data produced in different countries and laboratories (see section 6.3).

6.2.1 *Pharmaceutical agents*

The earliest testing protocols for reproductive toxicity were developed for pharmaceutical agents by the US Food and Drug Administration (FDA) in 1966. These protocols are based on a three-segment design that gives a fairly complete picture of the reproductive and developmental effects of a particular drug. Segment I is an overall evaluation of fertility and reproduction in which males and females (usually rats) are exposed prior to mating and females are also exposed throughout pregnancy and lactation. Segment II includes teratogenicity testing as well as outcomes such as growth alteration and mortality. It is carried out on a rodent and a non-rodent species. Dams are treated during the period of major organogenesis, and fetuses are examined in detail just before parturition. Segment III is a peri- and postnatal study, in which animals (usually rats) are treated from the end of major organogenesis through parturition and lactation. Effects on pup survival, growth and development are assessed. This approach was used for many years, with slight differences between the US/European guidelines and those recommended in Japan. Testing guidelines have been updated for pharmaceuticals (ICH, 1993) and for certain food additives and chemicals.

In 1994 and 1995, two jointly sponsored IPCS/OECD international workshops were held to try to harmonize the different approaches to reproductive and developmental toxicity risk assessment (IPCS, 1995; Chahoud et al., 1999). The focus of these workshops was to identify and discuss the areas of agreement and disagreement on approaches to reproductive and developmental toxicity risk assessment; once identified, proposals were made for research that could help resolve areas of disagreement and uncertainty. The workshop reports indicated a number of areas of agreement and several research needs. One of the research needs was harmonization of terminology. A glossary that helps address this issue with respect to terminology for structural abnormalities was recently published (Wise et al., 1997). In addition, an Atlas of Developmental Abnormalities in Common Laboratory Mammals was developed by the International Federation of Teratology Societies using the glossary. This document is available on the Internet (http://www.ifts-atlas.org).

6.2.2   Chemicals

Similar experimental protocols are used to test pesticides and food additives. Tests should cover both high-level acute and low-level long-term exposure; for environmental chemicals, there is greater need for study of long-term, low-level exposures. Protocols for testing long-term exposure (multigeneration studies, *in utero* toxicity tests) have been used since 1966. Guidelines include the US FDA (1970) guidelines for food additives and contaminants and the US EPA (1998a, 1998b, 1998c) and the OECD (1981a, 1983a, 1983b, 1996a) guidelines for pesticides and industrial chemicals. For non-food use pesticides, the strategy is generally to conduct a two-generation reproductive toxicity test (OECD, 2001b) and a prenatal developmental toxicity test (OECD, 2001a).

Food use pesticides and food additives are among the agents most exhaustively tested for reproductive toxicity, typically employing prenatal and multigeneration reproductive toxicity tests. A developmental neurotoxicity study may be included if there is concern about potential effects on the developing nervous system. Such a study may be conducted as a "stand-alone" or as part of a multigeneration reproduction study. Criteria for selecting agents for developmental neurotoxicity testing have been proposed and include evidence for CNS malformations, neuropathology in adults, neurotoxicity in adults and other signs of developmental toxicity.

Several factors are considered in developing specific testing requirements for industrial chemicals, including tonnage of chemical produced, uses of the chemical, potential for human exposure and structural analogy to toxic chemicals. These factors can be used as a basis for an appropriate testing strategy. Thus, a chemical intermediate produced only in a closed reactor system would have little or no mandated testing, because the probability of its release into the environment or of human exposure to the chemical is very low.

The European Union has adopted a tiered testing approach for new chemicals. This approach requires stepwise increases in detailed testing and evaluation when known factors (such as tonnage) warrant such increased testing. For those compounds that are produced at less than 1 tonne per annum and for which there are no structural or other alerts, no formal additional testing is required. As tonnage increases, the authorities require an OECD single-generation reproduction study. Results from this and other toxicity evaluations could then trigger the need for a prenatal toxicity test in one species. When the tonnage and additional information indicating potential effects increase, a multigeneration study would be required, together with the possibility of a prenatal study in a second species. When results are suggestive of, or demonstrate, adversity, then detailed clarification is required using more complex standard protocol studies or other investigative treatment and assessment regimes. For agents produced in high tonnage or for which extensive human exposure is known or expected, the normal testing strategy is to conduct a multigeneration reproduction study in conjunction with prenatal toxicity testing in two species, most frequently the rat and rabbit. This flexible strategy is a pragmatic approach to testing (EC, 1994). The testing strategy is currently being updated to include consideration of the revisions of the existing OECD guidelines (i.e., OECD, 2001a, 2001b) and the proposed draft OECD guideline for developmental neurotoxicity (OECD, 1999c).

Recent legislation in the USA (the Safe Drinking Water Act Amendments and the Food Quality Protection Act; US EPA, 1996a) mandated that the US EPA must develop a screening and testing strategy for hormonally active agents using approved and validated test methodology (US EPA, 1998d). The OECD is also implementing collaborative activities on validation of test methods for endocrine disrupters (OECD, 1999a, 1999b). The precise content of the screening battery and how the data will be used are currently the subjects of intense debate.

6.3 Sources of data on reproductive toxicity

Reproductive toxicity can be assessed using data from a variety of sources, including studies designed for other purposes (Chapin et al., 1998). Such data are often useful because they provide broader assessment of reproductive toxicity, and it is valuable to integrate the information from different sets of data. For example, it is common to perform histological evaluation of the reproductive organs in general toxicity studies (i.e., repeated-dose 28-day or 90-day studies). These frequently performed studies often provide the first indication of the potential reproductive toxicity of a compound (e.g., decrease in organ weight, histopathology). General toxicity studies may, however, use different doses or a different method of dosing than reproductive and developmental toxicity studies.

A number of specific protocols have been developed to evaluate reproductive toxicity. These vary from complex *in vivo* studies with multiple end-points to more simple *in vitro* studies using cells or embryos (ECETOC, 1989). The major *in vivo* study protocols are the single- and multigeneration reproductive studies (OECD, 1983a, 1983b; EC, 1996; US EPA, 1998a) and the prenatal toxicity study (US FDA, 1966; US EPA, 1998b; OECD, 2001a).

Two additional protocols have received international endorsement as screens for reproductive and developmental toxicity (OECD, 1995, 1996b). These *in vivo* protocols were specifically designed for prioritization of future investigations and not as specific "stand-alone" studies for risk assessment purposes. Their original intent was for gathering information on chemicals for which no information was available. These protocols are more limited in scope and duration than the generally accepted protocols; therefore, a positive finding is likely to indicate toxicity and warrant further study. In contrast, a negative finding is insufficient and inconclusive with respect to potential reproductive toxicity. Alternative protocols include continuous breeding studies (Lamb, 1985) and the alternative reproductive test (Gray et al., 1988). In a few cases, studies to evaluate developmental neurotoxicity or other postnatal functions may have been conducted, and these can provide a more complete evaluation of potential developmental effects. In addition to the standard guideline studies, data from experimental studies on mechanisms of action, etc., can provide useful data for consideration in the risk assessment process.

These reproductive toxicity protocols and guidelines have improved our ability to assess potential adverse effects, but there is still considerable difficulty in interpreting studies using different end-points. A workshop convened by the International Life Sciences Institute (ILSI, 1999) identified the need for guidance on how to interpret data from various reproductive toxicity tests and how this applies to human health risk assessment. Workshop participants agreed that an integrated approach was essential and that biological plausibility should dictate the validity of any given observation.

6.4   Hazard identification

Hazard identification is the first stage in hazard assessment or risk assessment, which consists of identifying substances of concern and the adverse effects they may have on target systems under certain conditions of exposure (OECD/IPCS, 2001).

The purpose of hazard identification is to evaluate the weight of evidence for adverse effects in humans based on assessment of all available data, ranging from observations in humans and animal data to an analysis of mechanisms of action and structure–activity relationships. Each source of information has its advantages and limitations, which determine the "weight" of that evidence; collectively, the evidence permits a scientific judgement as to whether the chemical can cause adverse effects.

A "weight of evidence" approach to assessing reproductive toxicity requires rigorous evaluation of all available data. However, often only limited information is available, and default assumptions must be made because of uncertainties in understanding mechanisms, dose–response relationships at low dose levels and human exposure patterns. Several of these assumptions are basic to the extrapolation of toxicity data from animals to humans, while others are specific to reproductive toxicity. The general default assumptions for reproductive toxicity stated in the IPCS (1995) report are summarized as follows:

■   An animal reproductive effect is assumed to be predictive of a potential human reproductive effect, although the precise manifestations may not be the same. This assumption is based on comparisons of data for agents that are known to cause human reproductive toxicity (Thomas, 1981; Meistrich, 1982; Nisbet & Karch, 1983; Kimmel et al., 1984; Hemminki & Vineis, 1985; Kimmel & Gaylor, 1988; Working, 1988; Newman et al., 1993).

■   In the absence of information on the most appropriate species, it is assumed that the most sensitive species is the most appropriate. This is because, for the majority of agents known to cause human reproductive toxicity, humans appear to be as sensitive as or more sensitive than the most sensitive species tested, based on studies that determined dose on a body weight or air concentration basis

(Thomas, 1981; Nisbet & Karch, 1983; Kimmel et al., 1984, 1990; Hemminki & Vineis, 1985; Working, 1988; Newman et al., 1993).

■ In the absence of specific information on both sexes, it is assumed that a chemical demonstrated to cause effects on sexual function and fertility in one sex may cause similar effects in the other sex. This assumption is based on the fact that (1) for most agents, the nature of the testing and the data available are limited, reducing confidence that the potential for toxicity to both sexes and their offspring has been examined equally; and (2) many of the mechanisms controlling important aspects of reproductive system function are similar in males and females and therefore could be susceptible to the same agents. Specific information demonstrating a mechanistic difference between the sexes or sufficient testing showing no effect in one sex could negate this assumption.

■ In general, a threshold or non-linear dose–response relationship is assumed in the dose–response curve for reproductive toxicity. This is based on known homeostatic, compensatory or adaptive mechanisms that must be overcome before a toxic end-point is manifested and on the rationale that cells and organs of the reproductive system and the developing organism have some capacity to repair damage. However, in a population, background levels of toxic agents and pre-existing conditions may increase the sensitivity of some individuals. Thus, exposure to a toxic agent may increase risk of adverse effects for some, but not all, individuals within a population. Although a threshold may exist for end-points of reproductive toxicity, it usually is not feasible to distinguish empirically between a true threshold and a non-linear relationship.

6.5 Human studies

In principle, well documented observational and epidemiological studies provide the most relevant information on human health effects, since they avoid extrapolation from animals to humans. However, for new chemicals, human data will not be available, and the potential toxicity of the chemical is estimated using experimental studies. Also, human populations are heterogeneous and may be differentially susceptible to chemical-induced effects (IPCS, 1984, 1986a, 1986b, 1992, 1996, 1999). Exposure to chemicals often occurs in occupational settings, where exposure tends to be higher than in the general population; nevertheless, studies on occupational exposures have provided valuable data on both the reproductive toxicity of many chemicals and effective study designs (see Lindbohm, 1999). The reproductive toxicity data for humans are limited to only a few chemicals, but the database is rapidly expanding. Fundamentals of epidemiology studies are not addressed here, since they are discussed in textbooks and reviews (Moolgavkar, 1995; Rothman & Greenland, 1998). Guidelines for conducting environmental epidemiology studies have also been published.

"Human studies" include both epidemiological studies and other reports of individual cases or clusters of events. Typical epidemiological studies include (1) cohort studies in which groups are defined by exposure and health outcomes are examined; (2) case–referent studies in which groups are defined by health status and prior exposures are examined; (3) cross-sectional studies in which exposure and outcome are determined at the same time; and (4) ecological studies in which exposure is presumed based typically on residence. Greatest weight should be given to carefully designed epidemiological studies with more precise measures of exposure, because they can best evaluate exposure–response relationships (Weinberg & Wilcox, 1998; Krzyzanowski, 2000). This assumes that human exposure occurs in a broad enough dose range for observable differences in response to occur. Epidemiological studies in which exposure is inferred from occupational title or residence (e.g., some case–referent and all ecological studies) may contribute data for hazard characterization; however, these studies are of limited value for quantitative risk determination because of the typically broad categorical groupings. Recent advances have improved exposure data in ecological studies. For example, mapping of monitoring data (using a geographic information system) allows improvements in assignment of potential exposure, taking into account emission patterns, topology and meteorological patterns. In addition, some ecological studies have included collection of more detailed breakdowns of mixtures or measurement of biomarkers for some (or all) of the subjects, allowing improved estimation of exposure.

Reports of individual cases or clusters of events may be used to generate hypotheses of exposure–outcome associations, which can be confirmed with well designed epidemiological or laboratory studies. These reports of cases or clusters may support associations suggested by other human or test animal data, but cannot be used for risk assessment in the absence of additional data. Detailed analysis of epidemiology data often requires specific professional training in this area. Some general design considerations and examination of data from various types of reports or studies are briefly discussed below.

6.5.1 Criteria for establishing causality

The strengths and weaknesses of each study must be considered along with the potential for bias (Rothman & Greenland, 1998), paying particular attention to exposure data, criteria for definition of health outcome under study and the size of the study population. A set of standardized criteria for assessing the weight of evidence of causality has been developed (Hill, 1965; Susser, 1977). The statistical power of the study (i.e., the probability that the study will be able to demonstrate an effect) must be evaluated. For example, to score a recognized fetal loss, hundreds of pregnancies must be evaluated (Little et al., 1999).

Power can be enhanced by combining populations from several studies using a meta-analysis (Blair et al., 1995; Blettner et al., 1999). The combined analysis can increase confidence in the absence of risk for agents with negative findings. However, caution must be exercised in combining potentially dissimilar study groups.

If a study has negative findings, it should be carefully evaluated with respect to, for example, the power of the study, its concordance or discordance with other related studies, and differences or similarities in study design or end-points with related studies. Results of different studies can be evaluated by comparing statistical confidence intervals. Studies with lower power will tend to yield wider confidence intervals; the magnitude of the risks must be considered. Studies with similar risks are important even if statistical significance is not present in all studies.

6.5.2   *Potential bias in data collection*

Bias may result from study group selection or methods of data collection (Rothman & Greenland, 1998). Selection bias can occur when an individual's willingness to participate varies with certain characteristics relating to exposure or health status. In addition, selection bias may operate in the identification of subjects for study. For example, hospital records are often used to identify the study group for early pregnancy loss, and this will underascertain events, because women are not always hospitalized for these outcomes. Risk assessment will give more weight to a study in which a more complete list of pregnancies is obtained, such as collection of biological data (e.g., hCG measurements) of pregnancy status from study members. Hospital records contain more complete data on congenital malformations than do birth certificates and can be used for ascertainment purposes (Mackerprang et al., 1972; Snell et al., 1992). Sperm bank or fertility clinic data may also be successfully used for semen studies. Study subjects from either of these sources are preferentially selected, because semen donors are typically of proven fertility and men in fertility clinics are part of a subfertile couple who are actively trying to conceive. These factors should be considered and evaluated prior to use in risk assessment.

Studies of working women present the potential for additional bias, because some factors that influence employment status may also affect reproductive end-points. For example, because of child care responsibilities, women may terminate employment, as might women with a history of reproductive problems who wish to have children and are concerned about workplace exposures (Joffe, 1985; Lemasters & Pinney, 1989). Thus, retrospective studies of female exposure that do not include terminated female workers may be of limited use in risk assessment, because the level of risk for some of the outcomes is likely to be overestimated (Lemasters & Pinney, 1989).

Information bias can result from misclassification of characteristics of individuals or events identified for study. Recall bias, one type of information bias, may occur when respondents with specific exposures or outcomes recall information differently from those without the exposures or outcomes. Interview bias may result when the interviewer knows *a priori* the category of exposure (for cohort studies) or outcome (for case–referent studies) in which the respondent belongs. Use of highly structured questionnaires and "blinding" of the interviewer reduce the likelihood of such bias. Studies with lower likelihood of such bias should carry more weight in a risk assessment (Axelson, 1985; Stein & Hatch, 1987; Weinberg et al., 1994).

Data from any source may be prone to errors or bias. Bias can be difficult to assess; however, validation with an independent data source (e.g., vital or hospital records) or use of biomarkers of exposure or outcome, where possible, may help identify bias and increase confidence in the results of the study.

6.5.3 Collection of data on other risk factors, effect modifiers and confounders

Factors that may affect reproductive toxicity include such characteristics as age, smoking, alcohol or caffeine consumption, drug use and past reproductive history. Some subpopulations may have increased or decreased susceptibility due to genetic, acquired or developmental characteristics. Known and potential risk factors should be examined to identify confounders or effect modifiers. An effect modifier is a factor that alters exposure–response relationships. For example, age is an effect modifier if the risk associated with a given exposure changes with age (e.g., an exposure that changes semen quality in older but not younger men). A confounder is a variable that is a risk factor for the disease under study and is associated with the exposure under study, but is not a consequence of the exposure. A confounder can distort both the magnitude and direction of the measure of association between the exposure of interest and the outcome. For example, smoking can be associated with socioeconomic status and with level of fertility, so smoking may be a confounder for studies of these outcomes.

Both effect modifiers and confounders need to be controlled in the study design and/or analysis to improve the estimate of the effects of exposure. A more in-depth discussion of these issues has been previously published (see Epidemiology Workshop for the Interagency Regulatory Liaison Group, 1981; Kleinbaum et al., 1982; Rothman & Greenland, 1998). Statistical techniques are available to control for these factors, and their application and interpretation require careful consideration (Kleinbaum et al., 1982; Rothman & Greenland, 1998).

Studies that fail to account for these important factors should be given less weight in a risk assessment.

6.5.4 Examination of clusters, case reports or series

Cases or clusters of adverse reproductive effects are generally identified by the individuals involved or their physicians. Subfecundity is difficult to identify in both males and females because it may be hard to recognize and can be viewed as a non-event. Cultural norms may inhibit the reporting of impaired fecundity in men. In addition, adverse pregnancy outcomes as a result of paternal exposure have been less studied and so may be less readily recognized and identified than those resulting from maternal exposure. The first agent identified as causing male reproductive toxicity in humans, dibromochloropropane, was identified from study of a cluster of male subfecundity. It was recognized by virtue of an atypically high level of communication among the wives of the exposed male workers (Whorton et al., 1977, 1979; Biava et al., 1978).

Adverse effects identified in clusters and case reports of females have been, thus far, primarily adverse pregnancy outcomes, such as fetal loss and congenital malformations. Identification of other effects, such as subfertility/subfecundity or menstrual cycle disorders, may be more difficult, as noted above.

Case reports are useful to identify agents that may cause reproductive toxicity. They are probably of greatest use in suggesting topics for further investigation. Reports of clusters and case reports/series are best used in risk assessment in conjunction with strong laboratory data to support the conclusion that similar effects occur in test animals and in humans.

6.5.5 Community studies and surveillance programmes

Epidemiological data are often based on broad populations such as a community, a nationwide probability sample, registries or disease surveillance programmes (Savitz & Harlow, 1991; Scialli et al., 1997). Potential toxicants are also monitored in outdoor air, food, water and soil. These measurements can be used to calculate estimated exposure of humans through contact with their contaminated environment. However, such environmental measurements are difficult to link to critical periods of exposure for a given reproductive effect. Some studies are more detailed, evaluating routes of exposure via indoor air, house dust and occupational exposures on an individual basis (Selevan, 1991). Such environmental studies, relating individual exposure to health outcome, are less likely to misclassify exposure and thus should be more useful in risk assessment.

Community studies have some limitations; for example, it may not be possible to distinguish maternal and paternal effects, because both parents are likely to occupy the same home environment. In addition, relatively low exposure levels are likely in community and home environments, such that very large groups are needed for study. A number of case–referent studies have examined whether classes of parental occupation correlate with incidence of embryo/fetal loss (Silverman et al., 1985; McDonald et al., 1989; Lindbohm et al., 1991; Agnesi et al., 1997; Borja-Aburto et al., 1999), birth defects (Hemminki et al., 1980; Kwa & Fine, 1980; Papier, 1985; Blatter et al., 1996, 1997; Laumon et al., 1996; Bianchi et al., 1997; Cordier et al., 1997; Garcia et al., 1998; Lorente et al., 2000) and childhood cancer (Fabia & Thuy, 1974; Hemminki et al., 1981; Peters et al., 1981; Gardner et al., 1990; Gold & Sever, 1994; Arbuckle & Sever, 1999; Feychting et al., 2000) in certain communities or countries. In these reports, jobs were classified into broad categories based on the probability of certain types or levels of exposure. Such studies can identify topics for future study. However, because of the broad groupings of types or levels of exposure, these studies are not typically useful for risk assessment of a particular agent.

Surveillance programmes also exist in occupational settings. In this case, it may be possible to follow reproductive histories (including menstrual cycles) or semen evaluations to monitor reproductive effects of exposure. With adequate exposure information, these could yield very useful data for risk assessment. Reproductive histories are easier and less costly to collect than semen evaluations. Semen studies also may have limited response rates, thus reducing their representativeness. It is important to reassure workers that the data they provide for such programmes remain confidential and will not affect their employment status (Samuels, 1988; Lemasters, 1993; Lindbohm, 1999).

6.6 Evaluation of dose–response relationships

The evaluation of dose–response relationships is a critical component of hazard characterization (OECD, 1989; ECETOC, 1992; US EPA, 1997a; IPCS, 1999). Evidence for a dose–response relationship is an important criterion in establishing a toxic reproductive effect. It includes the evaluation of data from both human and laboratory animal studies. Because quantitative data on human dose–response relationships are infrequently available, the dose–response evaluation is usually based on the assessment of data from tests performed using laboratory animals. However, if data are available in humans with a sufficient range of doses, dose–response relationships in humans can also be evaluated.

The dose–response relationships for individual end-points, as well as for combinations of end-points, must be examined. Dose–response evaluations should consider the effects that competing risks between different end-points may have on outcomes observed at different exposure levels. For example, an agent might increase abnormal sperm morphology at a low dose, but might decrease total sperm count and decrease the relative proportion of abnormal sperm at higher doses. Similarly, malformation or decreased fetal weight might be observed at a low dose, but prenatal death and decrease in the proportion of malformed offspring might occur at a higher dose. Whenever possible, pharmacokinetic data should be used to determine the effective dose of the target organ.

When data on several species are available, the species most relevant to humans is the most appropriate for a dose–response evaluation. This choice is based on several factors, including comparable physiological, pharmacological, pharmacokinetic and pharmacodynamic processes; the adequacy of dosing; the appropriateness of the route of administration; and the end-points selected. However, information of this nature is often very limited, and no single laboratory animal species can be considered the best for predicting risk of reproductive toxicity to humans in all situations. In some cases, such as in the assessment of physiological parameters related to menstrual disorders, higher non-human primates are generally considered similar to humans. In the absence of a clearly most relevant species, data from the most sensitive species (i.e., the species showing a toxic effect at the lowest administered dose) are used, because, as mentioned above, humans are assumed to be as sensitive as the most sensitive animal species (Nisbet & Karch, 1983; Kimmel et al., 1984; Hemminki & Vineis, 1985; Working, 1988; Newman et al., 1993).

The evaluation of dose–response relationships includes the identification of effective dose levels as well as doses that are associated with low or no increased incidence of adverse effects compared with controls. Many studies identify either the lowest dose causing an adverse effect (lowest-observed-adverse-effect level, or LOAEL) or the no-observed-adverse-effect level (NOAEL) (Calabrese & Baldwin, 1994).

Generally, in studies that do not evaluate reproductive toxicity, only adult male and non-pregnant females are examined. Therefore, it is often unknown if pregnant females are particularly sensitive to an agent. In studies in which reproductive toxicity has been evaluated, the effective dose range should be identified for both reproductive and other forms of systemic toxicity and should be compared with the corresponding values from other adult toxicity data to determine if the pregnant or lactating female is more sensitive to an agent.

Studies should also evaluate the route of exposure, timing and duration of exposure, species specificity of effects and any pharmaco-kinetic or other considerations that might influence human exposure. Information should also be obtained as relevant from the health-related database.

For the developing organism, which changes rapidly and is vulner-able at a number of stages, it is assumed that a single exposure at a critical time in development can produce an adverse developmental effect (US EPA, 1991). Therefore, with inhalation exposures, the daily dose is usually not adjusted to a 24-h equivalent with developmental toxicity unless appropriate pharmacokinetic data are available. However, for other reproductive effects, daily doses by inhalation may be adjusted for duration of exposure (US EPA, 1996b). These differences need to be reviewed to determine the most appropriate approach.

6.6.1 Quantitative dose–response assessment

Quantitative dose–response assessment involves the determination of a NOAEL or benchmark dose (BMD) and low-dose estimation or extrapolation. Usually a non-linear (threshold) dose–response relationship at low dose levels is assumed unless a specific mode of action or pharmacodynamic data are available to indicate otherwise (IPCS, 1986c). If sufficient data on mode of action, underlying reproductive and developmental processes and pharmacokinetics/pharmacodynamics are available, a biologically based approach may be used to predict dose–response relationships at low exposure levels. At the present time, sufficient information is rarely available for this approach (see Shuey et al., 1994, for an example). Thus, a chemical-specific approach is used that incorporates information on the mode of action of a particular chemical and its pharmacokinetics. In most cases, however, data are available only on exposure level and associated adverse outcomes. In these instances, the dose–response analysis consists of evaluating the dose–response relationships within the observable range and determining the NOAEL, LOAEL or BMD, then using this information to calculate a low level of exposure (guidance or reference level) that is considered to be without appreciable risk (IPCS, 1994). This is typically done through the use of uncertainty factors applied to the NOAEL, LOAEL or BMD, but may also be done by low-dose extrapolation when data are available to support such an approach.

6.6.2 Determination of the NOAEL, LOAEL, BMD and guidance levels

As mentioned above, the NOAEL is the highest dose at which no adverse effects are detected, and the LOAEL is the lowest dose at which an adverse reproductive effect is detected compared with the appropriate controls. These doses are often identified based on statistical differences from controls, but can be determined by examining the trend in response and certain biological considerations, such as rarity of the effect. Evidence for biological significance can be strengthened by supporting evidence such as mode of action or biochemical response at low exposure. The existence of a NOAEL does not indicate that a threshold or non-linear dose–response relationship exists below the observable range; it only defines the highest level of exposure at which no significant adverse effect is observed under the conditions of the study.

Mathematical modelling of the dose–response relationship is an alternative approach to quantify the estimated response within the experimental range. This approach can be used to determine the BMD or benchmark concentration (BMC) for inhalation exposure, which can be used in place of the LOAEL or NOAEL (Crump, 1984). The BMD (used here for either BMD or BMC) is defined as the lower confidence limit on a dose that produces a particular level of response (e.g., 1%, 5%, 10%) and has several advantages over the LOAEL or NOAEL (Kimmel & Gaylor, 1988; Kimmel, 1990; US EPA, 1995; IPCS, 1999). For example, (1) the BMD approach uses all of the data in fitting a model instead of only data indicating the LOAEL or NOAEL; (2) by fitting all of the data, the BMD approach takes into account the slope of the dose–response curve; (3) the BMD takes into account variability in the data; and (4) the BMD is not limited to one experimental dose. Calculation and use of the BMD approach are described in a US EPA (1995) document. Guidance for application of BMD in the risk assessment process is currently being developed (US EPA, 1996c), and software for calculating the BMD is available on the Internet (http://www.epa.gov/ncea/bmds.htm).

Several approaches to calculating BMDs for prenatal developmental toxicity data have been evaluated (Allen et al., 1994a, 1994b; Faustman et al., 1994; Kavlock et al., 1995). These studies apply several dose–response models, both generic and developmental toxicity-specific models, to a large number of standard developmental toxicity studies with dosing throughout the period of major organogenesis (or, in some cases, throughout pregnancy). These studies show that such models can be used successfully with prenatal developmental toxicity data. In a study of the proportion of implants or offspring affected per litter, the BMD for a 5% excess risk above controls corresponded on average to the NOAEL. Variables such as intralitter correlation and litter size appeared to enhance the fit of the developmental toxicity-specific models. BMDs from quantal data (i.e., the number of litters affected) for a 10% excess risk corresponded on average closely to the NOAEL. Various models were also applied to fetal weight data, and approaches for determining BMDs for continuous data were established (Kavlock et al., 1995). BMDs similar to the NOAEL were also obtained using several different definitions of difference between experimental and control values. A workshop was recently held on the criteria for application of the BMD concept. One of the conclusions reached at the time of that workshop was that sufficient information was available to begin using the BMD approach for developmental toxicity (Barnes et al., 1995).

The NOAEL, LOAEL or BMD approach can be used to calculate a guidance or reference level of exposure below which no adverse effects above background would be expected. These guidance levels include reference dose (RfD), acceptable daily intake (ADI) and tolerable daily intake (TDI).

6.6.3 *Low-dose estimation/extrapolation*

In quantitative dose–response analysis, a non-linear dose–response relationship (threshold) is generally assumed for reproductive toxicity (and for many other health effects), unless the mode of action of the agent is genotoxic. Because of the threshold assumption, it is not usually appropriate to use mathematical models to extrapolate to low doses for reproductive toxicity. Instead, a guidance value is set based on oral, dermal or inhalation data for chronic exposure. This approach does not estimate risk at a particular dose level, so when exposure occurs at levels above the guidance value, there is no way to estimate risk at that dose level; this is viewed as a significant disadvantage. Because of the short duration of most studies of developmental toxicity and the fact that a single exposure may be sufficient to produce a developmental effect, a separate guidance value for developmental toxicity (e.g., an RfD_{DT} or RfC_{DT}) can be determined. However, this procedure is not followed when developmental toxicity is the "critical effect," i.e., the effect at the lowest dose level.

The guidance/reference value is derived by dividing the NOAEL or BMD for the critical effect by uncertainty factors that account for such things as animal to human extrapolation, variations in sensitivity within the human population, lack of a NOAEL and various deficiencies in the database. The uncertainty factor is unique for a given agent, and considerable scientific judgement is required to arrive at a satisfactory value for this factor. Where there are adequate toxicokinetic or toxicodynamic data, default values can be replaced with compound-specific adjustments. As part of the IPCS project on the Harmonization of Approaches to the Assessment of Risk from Exposure to Chemicals, a document has been prepared to provide guidance on the use of such data to replace default uncertainty factors (IPCS, 2001b).

6.7 Exposure assessment

Exposure assessment describes the magnitude, duration, frequency and route of exposure to the agent of interest (WHO, 1999). The OECD/IPCS project on the harmonization of hazard/risk assessment terminology (OECD/IPCS, 2001) has defined exposure assessment as consisting of a quantitative and qualitative analysis of the amount of a chemical or biological agent, including its derivatives, that may be present in a given environment and the inference of the possible consequences it may have for a given population of particular concern. This information may come from hypothetical values, models or actual experimental values, including ambient environmental sampling results. Guidelines for exposure assessment have been published (US EPA, 1992) and will not be discussed in detail here; rather, issues important to reproductive toxicity risk assessment are addressed. One important issue is the necessary assumption that exposure of almost any segment of the population is important in relation to reproductive toxicity. Other issues include the route of exposure, absorption, persistence, pharmacokinetic properties of the chemical and the potential for multiple sources of exposure.

For reproductive/developmental toxicity, the routes by which the fetus could be exposed are critical and can depend on maternal absorption, distribution, metabolism and placental transfer of the chemical or its metabolite.

For all studies of reproductive toxicity, it is crucial to define the exposure that produces the effect. Preconceptional exposures of either parent and *in utero* exposures have been associated with common outcomes (e.g., fetal loss, malformation, low birth weight and infertility or subfertility). These exposures, plus postnatal exposure via breast milk, food and the environment, can also be associated with postnatal developmental effects (e.g., changes in growth or in behavioural and cognitive function). Infants and young children may be disproportionately exposed to pesticides because they eat more food and drink more water per kilogram than adults. In addition, they spend more time playing on the floor at home, in schools and in day care centres. Carpet can be a reservoir for toxicants (e.g., pesticides and lead dust), and the air near the floor may have a higher concentration of airborne toxicants (e.g., mercury from latex paints). Children also spend more time playing outside in grass and soil where contaminants are likely to be present. Spray can drift from nearby agricultural areas, and some children are exposed when they go to agricultural fields with their parents. Default values have been used for estimating sources of exposure to children (US NRC, 1993; WHO, 1999).

Breast-feeding is a major source of postnatal exposure to lipophilic agents, which can accumulate in breast milk. After several months of breast-feeding, the contaminant concentration in a child's adipose tissue is approximately equal to the concentration in the mother's tissue (Sonawane, 1995). Several potentially toxic agents have been found in breast milk, including pesticides (e.g., DDT and DDE, dieldrin, aldrin, endrin and HCB), other persistent organohalogens (e.g., dioxins, dibenzofurans, PCBs and polybrominated biphenyls, or PBBs) and heavy metals (e.g., lead, cadmium and mercury). Unlike the other agents, the heavy metals are not associated with milk fat. Data also suggest that stored lead may be mobilized from a mother's bone along with calcium during pregnancy and excreted in milk during lactation (Silbergeld et al., 1988; Silbergeld, 1991; Watson et al., 1993). Concerns over toxic exposures and breast-feeding are difficult to resolve due to the great benefits of breast-feeding (e.g., immunological, plus physical and psychological well-being). In general, with the exception of high maternal exposures (e.g., accidental poisonings), medical professionals emphasize the benefits of breast-feeding. This is an area that deserves more attention in the future.

The susceptibility of elderly men and women to chemical insults has not been well studied. Although the ability to procreate may no longer be a major health concern with elderly individuals, other biological functions maintained by the gonads (e.g., hormone production) are of significance (Walker, 1986). An exposure assessment should characterize the likelihood of exposure of several different subgroups (embryo or fetus, neonate, juvenile, young adult, older adult), and the risk assessment should address the susceptibility of different age groups as much as possible (IPCS, 1992).

Exposure can be ascertained at a particular point in time, a "critical window," or can reflect cumulative exposure. Each approach makes assumptions about the underlying relationship between exposure and outcome. For example, a cumulative exposure measure assumes that total exposure is important, with a greater probability of effect with greater total exposure or body burden. A dichotomous exposure measure (ever exposed versus never exposed) assumes an irreversible effect of exposure. Models that define exposure during a critical window assume that only the exposure during that time period is important. The appropriate exposure model depends on the biological processes affected and the nature of the chemical under study. Thus, a cumulative or dichotomous exposure model will be appropriate if injury occurs in cells that cannot be replaced or repaired (e.g., oocytes); a concurrent exposure model will be more appropriate when the chemical affects cells that are generated continually (e.g., spermatozoa) or when a critical window exists in prenatal or early postnatal development. Timing of exposure during gestation or early postnatal development is a key factor in the specific outcomes observed.

6.8 Risk characterization

Risk characterization is the qualitative and/or quantitative estimation, including attendant uncertainties, of the severity and probability of known and potential adverse effects of a substance in a given population; it is based on hazard identification, dose–response assessment and exposure assessment (OECD/IPCS, 2001), as described above.

Risk characterization integrates all available data. Table 4 summarizes guidance issued by the US EPA for developing chemical-specific risk characterization for reproductive effects.

6.8.1 Characterization of the database

The risk characterization should summarize the kinds of data brought together in the analysis and the reasoning on which the assessment is based. The description should convey the major strengths and weaknesses of the assessment that arise from availability of data and the current limits of our understanding of the mechanism of toxicity. A general format for summarizing toxicological data was developed by Moore et al. (1995), and a process based on this format was adopted by the IPCS Working Group on the Harmonization of Risk Assessment for Reproductive and Developmental Toxicity (IPCS, 1995). This process will also be used by the NTP's Center for the Evaluation of Risks to Human Reproduction (http://cerhr.niehs.nih.gov). This process is intended to be transparent so that enough detail is provided for the

Table 4. Guide for developing chemical-specific risk characterizations for reproductive effects[a]

I. Characterization of hazard

A. What is (are) the key toxicological study (or studies) that provides the basis for health concerns for reproductive effects?
    • How good is the key study?
    • Are the data from laboratory or field studies? In a single or multiple species?
    • What adverse reproductive end-points were observed, and what is the basis for the critical effect?
    • Describe other studies that support this finding.
    • Discuss any valid studies that conflict with this finding.

B. Besides the reproductive effect observed in the key study, are there other health end-points of concern? What are the significant data gaps?

C. Discuss available epidemiological or clinical data. For epidemiological studies:
    • What types of data were used (e.g., ecological, case–control or cohort studies, or case reports or series)?
    • Describe the degree to which exposures were described.
    • Describe the degree to which confounding factors were accounted for.
    • Describe the degree to which other causal factors were excluded.

D. How much is known about how (through what biological mechanism) the chemical produces adverse reproductive effects?
    • Discuss relevant studies of mechanisms of action or metabolism.
    • Does this information aid in the interpretation of the toxicity data?
    • What are the implications for potential adverse reproductive effects?

E. Comment on any non-positive data in animals or people, and whether these data were considered in the hazard characterization.

F. If adverse health effects have been observed in wildlife species, characterize such effects by discussing the relevant issues as in A through E above.

G. Summarize the hazard characterization and discuss the significance of each of the following:
    • Confidence in conclusions
    • Alternative conclusions that are also supported by the data
    • Significant data gaps
    • Highlights of major assumptions.

Table 4 (contd).

II. Characterization of dose–response

A. What data were used to develop the dose–response curve? Would the
    result have been significantly different if based on a different data set?
    • If laboratory animal data were used:
      – Which species were used? Most sensitive, average of all species,
        or other?
      – Were any studies excluded? Why?
    • If epidemiological data were used:
      – Which studies were used? Only positive studies, all studies, or
        some other combination?
      – Were any studies excluded? Why?
      – Was a meta-analysis performed to combine the epidemiological
        studies? What approach was used?

B. Was a model used to develop the dose–response curve, and, if so,
    which one?
    • What rationale supports this choice?
    • Is chemical-specific information available to support this approach?
    • How was the RfD/RfC (or the acceptable range) calculated?
    • What assumptions and uncertainty factors were used?
    • What is the confidence in the estimates?

C. Discuss the route, level and duration of exposure observed, as
    compared with expected human exposures.
    • Are the available data from the same route of exposure as the
      expected human exposures? If not, are pharmacokinetic data
      available to extrapolate across route of exposure?
    • How far does one need to extrapolate from the observed data to
      environmental exposures (one to two orders of magnitude? multiple
      orders of magnitude)? What is the impact of such an extrapolation?

D. If adverse health effects have been observed in wildlife species,
    characterize dose–response information using the process outlined in
    A–C.

III. Characterization of exposure

A. What are the most significant sources of environmental exposure?
    • Are there data on sources of exposure from different media?
    • What is the relative contribution of different sources of exposure?
    • What are the most significant environmental pathways for
      exposure?

B. Describe the populations that were assessed, including the general
    population, highly exposed groups and highly susceptible groups.

C. Describe the basis for the exposure assessment, including any
    monitoring, modelling or other analyses of exposure distributions, such
    as Monte Carlo or kriging.

Table 4 (contd).

D.   What are the key descriptors of exposure?
- Describe the (range of) exposures to: "average" individuals, "high-end" individuals, general population, high-exposure group(s), children, susceptible populations, males, females (non-pregnant, pregnant, lactating).
- How was the central tendency estimate developed?
- What factors and/or methods were used in developing this estimate?
- How was the high-end estimate developed?
- Is there information on highly exposed subgroups? Who are they? What are their levels of exposure? How are they accounted for in the assessment?

E.   Is there reason to be concerned about cumulative or multiple exposures because of biological, ethnic, racial or socioeconomic reasons?

F.   If adverse reproductive effects have been observed in wildlife species, characterize wildlife exposure by discussing the relevant issues as in A through E above.

G.   Summarize exposure conclusions and discuss the following:
- Results of different approaches, i.e., modelling, monitoring, probability distributions
- Limitations of each, and the range of most reasonable values
- Confidence in the results obtained, and the limitations to the results.

ª Taken from US EPA (1996b).

reader to understand the basis for decisions and to develop alternative decisions when appropriate. The process can be modified to suit particular circumstances, and two examples can be found in Moore (1995, 1997). The following statement is the format recommended by Moore et al. (1995) and Moore (1997) for summarizing the risk characterization of a particular agent:

> There is [*sufficient, limited, insufficient*] evidence in [*humans and/or animals*] that [*chemical/agent*] [*does or does not*] cause [*reproductive toxicity, effects on sexual function and fertility in males/females, developmental toxicity*] when exposure is [*route, dose range, timing, duration*]. Relationship to adult toxicity stated. The data are [*relevant, assumed relevant, irrelevant*] to humans. The rationale for all decisions must be stated.

6.8.2 Risk descriptors

There are a number of ways to describe risks for reproductive toxicity. The first is related to interindividual variability, which is the range of variability in response to an agent in a given population and the potential for existence of highly sensitive or susceptible groups within that population. A default assumption is that the most sensitive individual in the population will be no more than 10-fold more sensitive than the average individual; thus, a default 10-fold uncertainty factor is often applied in calculating the RfD or RfC to account for this potential difference. When data are available on highly sensitive or susceptible subpopulations, their risk can be characterized separately or by using more accurate factors to account for the differences. When data are not available to indicate differential susceptibility among reproductive phases or between males and females, all stages of reproduction are usually assumed to be highly sensitive or susceptible. Certain age subpopulations can sometimes be identified as more sensitive because of critical periods for exposure — for example, pregnant or lactating women, infants, children, adolescents or the elderly. In general, not enough is understood about how to identify sensitive subpopulations without specific data on each agent, although it is known that factors such as nutrition, personal habits, quality of life, pre-existing disease, race, ethnic background or other genetic factors may predispose some individuals to the reproductive toxicity of various agents.

The second important descriptor is concerned with population exposure. For example, what portion of the population exceeds the RfD/RfC, ADI or other guidance value? In some cases, the focus is on highly exposed individuals. These are individuals who are more highly exposed because of occupation, residential location, behaviour or other factors. For example, children are more likely than adults to be exposed to agents deposited in dust or soil either indoors or outside, both because of the time children spend crawling or playing on the floor or ground and because of the mouthing behaviour of young children. The inherent sensitivity of children may also vary with age, so that both sensitivity and exposure must be considered to characterize their risk. If population data are absent, various scenarios can be assumed for high-level exposure using upper-percentile or judgement-based values. This approach must be used with caution, however, to avoid over-estimation of exposure.

The third descriptor that is sometimes used to characterize risk is the margin of exposure (MOE). The MOE is the ratio of the NOAEL (or BMD) from the most appropriate or sensitive species to the estimated level of human exposure from all potential sources.

Considerations for the acceptability of the MOE are similar to those for the uncertainty factor used to calculate the RfD, RfC or other reference values from the NOAEL or BMD. The MOE has been calculated from reproductive toxicity data for several chemicals. Examples include dinoseb (US EPA, 1986), lithium (Moore, 1995) and boric acid and borax (Moore, 1997). In the case of dinoseb, the MOEs were very low, in some cases less than one, indicating toxicity in the animal studies at levels to which people are exposed. This information on dinoseb led to an emergency suspension of use of this pesticide in the USA in 1986 and ultimately led to its removal from the market (Kimmel & Kimmel, 1994, 1996).

Reproductive risk descriptors are intended to address variability of risk within the population and the overall adverse impact on the population. In particular, differences between high-end and central tendency estimates reflect variability in the population but not the scientific uncertainty inherent in the risk estimates. There is uncertainty in all estimates of risk, including reproductive risk. These uncertainties can result from measurement uncertainties, modelling uncertainties and assumptions made due to incomplete data. Risk assessments should address the impact of each of these uncertainties on confidence in the estimated reproductive risk values.

Both qualitative and quantitative evaluations of uncertainty provide useful information in a risk assessment. The techniques of quantitative uncertainty analysis are evolving rapidly. An approach was recently proposed for estimating distribution of uncertainty in non-cancer risk assessments (Baird et al., 1996).

6.9   Summary

This chapter summarizes the risk assessment strategies for reproductive toxicity, including effects on sexual function and fertility and on developmental toxicity. Guidance on principles and specific protocols for risk assessment for reproductive toxicity has been published elsewhere. It is evident that assumptions must be made in the risk assessment process because of gaps in knowledge about underlying biological processes and in extrapolating data from one species to another. The processes of hazard characterization, quantitative dose–response analysis and exposure assessment must be integrated in the final characterization of risk, which must be evaluated and summarized. The approaches described in this chapter can be applied to thoroughly evaluate the potential for reproductive risk as a result of exposure. Although a number of advances have been made in the approaches for reproductive risk assessment, there are still many gaps in the knowledge base and a need for research to fill those gaps.

REFERENCES

Aafjes JH, Vels JM, & Schenck E (1980) Fertility of rats with artificial oligozoospermia. J Reprod Fertil, **58**: 345–351.

Adamopoulos DA, Pappa A, Nicopoulou S, Andreou E, Karametzanis M, Mievhopoulos J, Deglianni V, & Simon M (1996) Seminal volume and total sperm number trends in men attending subfertility clinics in the greater Athens area during the period 1977–1993. Hum Reprod, **11**: 1936–1941.

Adams J & Buelke-Sam J (1981) Behavioral assessment of the postnatal animal: Testing and methods development. In: Kimmel CA & Buelke-Sam J ed. Developmental toxicology. New York, Raven Press, pp 233–258.

Adashi EY, Resnick CE, Hernandez ER, Svoboda ME, & Van Wyk JJ (1989) Potential relevance of insulin-like growth factor 1 to ovarian physiology: from basic to clinical application. Endocr Rev, **7**: 94.

Agnesi R, Valentini F, & Mastrangelo G (1997) Risk of spontaneous abortion and maternal exposure to organic solvents in the shoe industry. Int Arch Occup Environ Health, **69**: 311–316.

Akre O, Cnattingius S, Bergstrom R, Kvist U, Trichopoulos D, & Ekbom A (1999a) Human fertility does not decline: evidence from Sweden. Fertil Steril, **71**: 1066–1069.

Akre O, Lipworth L, Cnattingius S, Sparen P, & Ekbom A (1999b) Risk factor patterns for cryptorchidism and hypospadias. Epidemiology, **10**: 364–369.

Alder S & Zbinden G (1977) Methods for the evaluation of physical, neuromuscular and behavioural development of rats in early postnatal life. In: Neubert D, Merker H-J, & Kwasigroch TE ed. Methods in prenatal toxicology. Stuttgart, Georg Thieme, pp 175–185.

Alexandrov VA (1976) Some results and prospects of transplacental carcinogenesis studies. Neoplasma, **23**(3): 285–299.

Allan BB, Brant R, Seidel JE, & Jarrell JF (1997) Declining sex ratios in Canada. Can Med Assoc J, **156**: 37–41.

Allen BC, Kavlock RJ, Kimmel CA, & Faustman EM (1994a) Dose–response assessment for developmental toxicity: II. Comparison of generic benchmark dose estimates with NOAELs. Fundam Appl Toxicol, **23**: 487–495.

Allen BC, Kavlock RJ, Kimmel CA, & Faustman EM (1994b) Dose–response assessment for developmental toxicity: III. Statistical models. Fundam Appl Toxicol, **23**: 496–509.

Allenby G, Foster PMD, & Sharpe RM (1991) Evaluation of the changes in the secretion of immunoreactive inhibin by adult rat seminiferous tubules *in vitro* as an indicator of early toxicant action on spermatogenesis. Fundam Appl Toxicol, **16**: 710–724.

Alm H, Tiemann U, & Torner H (1996) Influence of organochlorine pesticides on development of mouse embryos *in vitro*. Reprod Toxicol, **10**: 321–326.

Amann RP (1970) Sperm production rates. In: Johnson AD, Gomes WR, & Vandemark NL ed. The testis. New York, Academic Press, pp 433–482.

Amann RP (1981) A critical review of methods for evaluation of spermatogenesis from seminal characteristics. J Androl, **2**: 37–58.

American Academy of Pediatrics Committee on Drugs (1994) The transfer of drugs and other chemicals into human milk. Pediatrics, **93**: 137–150.

Anderson D (2000) Does paternal exposure result in congenital abnormalities in offspring and a predisposition to cancer? In: Anderson D, Karakaya AE, & Sram RJ ed. Human monitoring after environmental and occupational exposure to chemical and physical agents. Amsterdam, IOS Press, pp 151–160 (NATO Science Series).

Anderson D, Edwards AJ, Brinkworth MH, & Hughes JA (1996) Male-mediated F1 effects in mice exposed to 1,3-butadiene. Toxicology, **113**: 120–127.

Anderson D, Edwards AJ, & Brinkworth MH (1998) A comparison of male-mediated effects in rats and mice exposed to 1,3-butadiene. Mutat Res, **397**: 77–84.

Ankley G, Milhaich E, Stahl R, Tillitt D, Colborn T, McMaster S, Miller R, Bantle J, Campbell P, Denslow N, Dickerson R, Folmar L, Fry M, Giesy G, Gray LE, Guiney P, Hutchinson T, Kennedy S, Kramer V, LeBlanc G, Mayes M, Nimrod A, Patino R, Peterson R, Purdy R, Ringer R, Thomas P, Touart L, Van Der Kraak G, & Zacharewski T (1998) Overview of a workshop on screening methods for detecting potential (anti-)estrogenic/androgenic chemicals in wildlife. Environ Toxicol Chem, **17**: 68–87.

Antich M, Fabian E, Sarquella J, & Bassas L (1995) Effect of testicular damage induced by cryptorchidism on insulin-like growth factor 1 receptors in rat Sertoli cells. J Reprod Fertil, **104**: 267.

Apostoli P, Bellini A, Porru S, & Bisanti L (2000) The effect of lead on male fertility: a time to pregnancy (TTP) study. Am J Ind Med, **38**: 310–315.

Arai Y, Mori T, Suzuki Y, & Bern HA (1983) Long-term effects of perinatal exposure to sex steroids and diethylstilbestrol on the reproductive system of male mammals. Int Rev Cytol, **84**: 235–268.

Arbuckle T & Sever L (1999) Pesticide exposure and fetal death: a review of the epidemiologic literature. Crit Rev Toxicol, **28**: 2229–2270.

Armstrong DT & Dorrington JH (1976) Androgens augment FSH-induced progesterone secretion by cultured rat granulosa cells. Endocrinology, **99**: 1411.

Aschengrau A & Monson RR (1989) Paternal military service in Vietnam and risk of spontaneous abortion. J Occup Med, **31**: 618–623.

Ashby J & Odum J (1998) The importance of protocol design and data reporting to research on endocrine disruption. Environ Health Perspect, **106**(7): 315–316.

Auger J, Kunstmann JM, Csyglik F, & Jouannet P (1995) Decline in semen quality among fertile men in Paris during the past 20 years. N Engl J Med, **332**: 281–285.

Autrup H (2000) Genetic polymorphisms in human xenobiotica metabolizing enzymes as susceptibility factors in toxic response. Mutat Res, **464**(1): 65–76.

Axelson O (1985) Epidemiologic methods in the study of spontaneous abortions: Sources of data, methods, and sources of error. In: Hemminki K, Sorsa M, & Vainio H ed. Occupational hazards and reproduction. Washington, DC, Hemisphere, pp 231–236.

Baird DD (1988) Using time-to-pregnancy data to study occupational exposures: methodology. Reprod Toxicol, **2**: 205–207.

Baird DD & Wilcox AJ (1985) Cigarette smoking associated with delayed conception. J Am Med Assoc, **253**: 2979–2983.

Baird DD, Wilcox AJ, & Weinberg CR (1986) Using time to pregnancy to study environmental exposures. Am J Epidemiol, **124**: 470–480.

Baird SJS, Cohen JT, Graham JD, Shlyakhter AI, & Evans JS (1996) Noncancer risk assessment: a probabilistic alternative to current practice. Hum Ecol Risk Assess, **2**: 79–102.

Baker TG (1963) A quantitative and cytological study of germ cells in human ovaries. Proc R Soc Lond Ser B, **158**: 417–433.

Baker TG (1982) Oogenesis and ovulation. In: Austin CR & Short RV ed. Germ cells and fertilization, 2nd ed. Vol. 1. Cambridge, Cambridge University Press, p 17.

Barlow SM & Sullivan FM (1975) Behavioural teratology. In: Berry CL & Poswillo DE ed. Teratology: Trends and applications. Berlin, Springer-Verlag, pp 103–120.

Barnes DG, Daston GP, Evans JS, Jarabek AM, Kavlock RJ, Kimmel CA, Park C, & Spitzer HL (1995) Benchmark dose workshop: criteria for use of a benchmark dose to estimate a reference dose. Regul Toxicol Pharmacol, **21**: 296–306.

Baukloh V, Bohnet HG, Trapp M, Heaschen W, Feichtinger W, & Kemeter P (1987) Biocides in human follicular fluid. Ann NY Acad Sci, **442**: 240–250.

Beach FA (1979) Animal models for human sexuality. In: Sex, hormones, and behavior. London, Elsevier/North-Holland, pp 113–143 (Ciba Foundation Symposium No. 62).

Bechter R & Terlouw GDC (1993) Strain differences in the control incidences of morphological abnormalities in the rat whole embryo culture. Toxicol In Vitro, **7**(Suppl 1): 281–284.

Beck F & Lloyd JB (1963) The preparation and teratogenic properties of pure trypan blue and its common contaminants. J Embryol Exp Morphol, **11**: 175–184.

Behringer RR (1995) The mullerian inhibitor and mammalian sexual development. Philos Trans R Soc Lond B Biol Sci, **350**(1333): 285–289.

Bellinger D (1995) Interpreting the literature on lead and child development: the neglected role of the "experimental system." Neurotoxicol Teratol, **17**(3): 201–212.

Bellinger D, Stiles K, & Needleman H (1992) Low-level lead exposure, intelligence and academic achievement: a long-term follow-up study. Pediatrics, **90**: 855–861.

Berendtson WE (1977) Methods for quantifying mammalian spermatogenesis: a review. J Anim Sci, **44**: 818–833.

Berman NG, Wang C, & Paulsen CA (1996) Methodological issues in the analysis of human sperm concentration data. J Androl, **17**: 68–73.

Bianchi F, Cianciulli D, Pierini A, & Seniori CA (1997) Congenital malformations and maternal occupation: a registry based case–control study. Occup Environ Med, **54**: 223–228.

Biava CG, Smuckler EA, & Whorton D (1978) The testicular morphology of individuals exposed to dibromochloropropane. Exp Mol Pathol, **29**: 448–458.

Bigelow PL, Jarrell J, Young MR, Keefe TJ, & Love EJ (1998) Association of semen quality and occupational factors: comparison of case–control analysis of continuous variables. Fertil Steril, **69**: 11–18.

Bishop JB & Kimmel CA (1997) Molecular and cellular mechanisms of early mammalian development: an overview of NIEHS/EPA developmental toxicity workshops. Reprod Toxicol, **11**: 285–291.

Blair A, Burg J, Foran J, Gibb H, Greenland S, Morris R, Raabe G, Savitz D, Teta J, & Wartenberg D (1995) Guidelines for application of meta-analysis in environmental epidemiology. ILSI Risk Science Institute. Regul Toxicol Pharmacol, **22**: 189–197.

Blatter BM, Roeleveld N, Zielhuis GA, Gabreels FJ, & Verbeek AL (1996) Maternal occupational exposure during pregnancy and the risk of spina bifida. Occup Environ Med, **53**: 80–86.

Blatter BM, Hermens R, Bakker M, Roeleveld N, Verbeek AL, & Zielhuis GA (1997) Paternal occupational exposure around conception and spina bifida in offspring. Am J Ind Med, **32**: 283–291.

Blettner M, Sauerbrei W, Schlehofer B, Scheuchenpflug T, & Friedenreich C (1999) Traditional reviews, meta-analyses and pooled analyses in epidemiology. Int J Epidemiol, **28**: 1–9.

Bloom AD (1981) Guidelines for reproductive studies in exposed human populations. Guideline for studies of human populations exposed to mutagenic and reproductive hazards. Report of Panel II. White Plains, New York, March of Dimes Birth Defects Foundation, pp 37–110.

Bobrow M & Grimbaldeston AH (2000) Medical genetics, the human genome project and public health. J Epidemiol Community Health, **54**(9): 645–649.

Bonde JP, Kold Jensen T, Brixen Larsen S, Abell A, Scheike T, Hjollund NH, Kolstad HA, Ernst E, Giwercman A, Skakkabaek NE, Keiding N, & Olsen J (1998a) Year of birth and sperm count in 10 Danish occupational studies. Scand J Work Environ Health, **24**: 407–413.

Bonde JP, Ernst E, Jensen TK, Hjollund NH, Kolstad HA, Henriksen TB, Scheike T, Giwercman A, Olsen J, & Skakkabaek NE (1998b) Relation between semen quality and fertility: a population-based study of 430 first-pregnancy planners. Lancet, **352**: 1172–1177.

Borja-Aburto VH, Hertz-Picciotto I, Rojas LM, Farias P, Rios C, & Blanco J (1999) Blood lead levels measured prospectively and risk of spontaneous abortion. Am J Epidemiol, **150**: 590–597.

Brent RL & Franklin JB (1960) Uterine vascular clamping: New procedure for the study of congenital malformations. Science, **132**: 89–91.

Brown N (1994) Normal development: Mechanisms of early embryogenesis. In: Kimmel CA & Buelke-Sam J ed. Development toxicology, 2nd ed. New York, Raven Press, pp 15–49.

Brown NA & Fabro S (1981) Quantitation of rat embryonic development *in vitro*: A morphological scoring system. Teratology, **24**: 65–78.

Buelke-Sam J, Kimmel CA, & Adams J ed. (1985) Proceedings of a conference on design considerations in screening for behavioral teratogens: Results of the collaborative behavioral teratology study. Neurobehav Toxicol Teratol, **7**(6): 537–789.

Burch TK, Macisco JJ, & Parker MP (1967) Some methodologic problems in the analysis of menstrual data. Int J Fertil, **12**: 67–76.

Burger HG & Findlay JK (1989) Potential relevance of inhibin to ovarian physiology. Semin Reprod Endocrinol, **7**: 69.

Bustos-Obregõn E, Courot M, Flechon JE, Hochereau-de-Reviers MT, & Holstein AF (1975) Morphological appraisal of gametogenesis. Spermatogenic process in mammals with particular reference to man. Andrologia, **7**: 141–163.

Calabrese EJ & Baldwin LA (1994) Improved method for detection of the NOAEL. Regul Toxicol Pharmacol, **19**: 48–50.

Campbell PM & Hutchinson TH (1998) Wildlife and endocrine disrupters: requirements for hazard identification. Environ Contam Toxicol, **17**: 127–135.

Carlson E, Giwercman A, Keiding N, & Skakkebaek NE (1992) Evidence for decreasing quality of semen during the past 50 years. Br Med J, **305**: 609–613.

Chahoud I, Buschmann J, Clark R, Druga A, Falke H, Faqi A, Hansen E, Heinrich-Hirsch B, Hellwig J, Lingk W, Parkinson M, Paumgarten FJR, Pfeil R, Platzek T, Scialli AR, Seed J, Stahlmann R, Ulbrich B, Wu Z, Yasuda M, Younes M, & Solecki R (1999) Classification terms in developmental toxicology: need for harmonization. Report of the second workshop on the terminology of developmental toxicology, Berlin, 27–28 August 1998. Reprod Toxicol, **13**(1): 77–82.

Challis JRG & Lye SJ (1994) Parturition. In: Knobil E & Neill JD ed. The physiology of reproduction, 2nd ed. New York, Raven Press, pp 985–1032.

Chapin RE & Heindel JJ ed. (1993) Methods in toxicology 3a: Male reproductive toxicology. San Diego, California, Academic Press.

Chapin RE, Filler RS, Gulati D, Heindel JJ, Katz DF, Mebus CA, Obasaju F, Perreault SD, Russel SR, Schrader S, Slott V, Sokol RZ, & Toth G (1992) Methods for assessing rat sperm motility. Reprod Toxicol **6**: 267–273.

Chapin RE, Sloane RA, & Haseman JK (1998) Reproductive endpoints in general toxicity studies: are they predictive? Reprod Toxicol **12**(4): 489–494.

Cheung YB, Low L, Osmond C, Barker D, & Karlberg J (2000) Fetal growth and early postnatal growth are related to blood pressure in adults. Hypertension, **36**(5): 795–800.

Christian MS (1993) Is there any place for nonmammalian *in vitro* tests? Reprod Toxicol, **7**(Suppl 1): 99–102.

Chubb C (1993) Male mouse sexual behaviour test. In: Chapin RE & Heindel JJ ed. Methods in toxicology 3a: Male reproductive toxicology. San Diego, California, Academic Press, pp 16–25.

Clarke DO, Duignan JM, & Welsch F (1992) 2-Methoxyacetic acid dosimetry–teratogenicity relationships in CD-1 mice exposed to 2-methoxyethanol. Toxicol Appl Pharmacol, 114: 77.

Cohen-Hubal EA, Sheldon LS, Burke JM, McCurdy TR, Berry MR, Rigas ML, Zartarian VG, & Freeman NC (2000) Children's exposure assessment: A review of factors influencing children's exposure, and the data available to characterize and assess that exposure. Environ Health Perspect, 108: 475–486.

Colborn T, Dumanowski D, & Myers JP (1996) Our stolen future. New York, Penguin Books Ltd.

Contreras HR & Bustos-Obregón E (1996) Effect of an organophosphorate insecticide on the testis, epididymis and preimplantational development and pregnancy outcome in mice. Int J Dev Biol, Suppl 1: 207S.

Contreras HR, Badilla J, & Bustos-Obregón E (1999) Morphofunctional disturbances of human sperm after incubation with organophosphate pesticides. Biocell, 23(2): 135–141.

Cooper RL & Kavlock RJ (1997) Endocrine disruptors and reproductive development: a weight-of-evidence overview. J Endocrinol, 152: 159–166.

Cooper RL & Walker RF (1979) Potential therapeutic consequences of age-dependent changes in brain physiology. Interdiscipl Topics Gerontol, 15: 54–76.

Cooper RL, Conn PM, & Walker RF (1980) Characterization of the LH surge in middle-aged female rats. Biol Reprod, 23: 611–615.

Cooper RL, Chadwick RW, Rehnberg GL, Goldman JM, Booth KC, Hein JF, & McElroy WK (1989) Effect of lindane on hormonal control of reproductive function in the female rat. Toxicol Appl Pharmacol, 99: 384–394.

Cordier S, Bergeret A, Goujard J, Ha MC, Ayme S, Bianchi F, Calzolari E, De Walle HE, Knill-Jones R, Candela S, Dale I, Dananche B, de Vigan C, Fevotte J, Kiel G, & Mandereau L (1997) Congenital malformation and maternal occupational exposure to glycol ethers. Occupational Exposure and Congenital Malformations Working Group. Epidemiology, 8: 355–363.

Crisp TM, Clegg ED, Cooper RL, Wood WP, Anderson DG, Baetcke KP, Hoffmann JL, Morrow MS, Rodier DJ, Schaeffer JE, Touart LW, Zeeman MG, & Patel YM (1998) Environmental endocrine disruption: an effects assessment and analysis. Environ Health Perspect, 1069(Suppl 1): 11–56.

Crofton KM (1990) Reflex modification and the detection of toxicant-induced auditory dysfunction. Neurotoxicol Teratol, 12(5): 461–468.

Crump KS (1984) A new method for determining allowable daily intakes. Fundam Appl Toxicol, 4: 854–871.

Csapo AI & Pulkkinen M (1978) Indispensability of the human corpus luteum in the maintenance of early pregnancy: Luteectomy evidence. Obstet Gynecol Surv, 33: 69-81.

Curtis KM, Savitz DA, Weinberg CR, & Arbuckle TE (1999) The effects of pesticide exposure on time to pregnancy. Epidemiology, 10: 112–117.

Daston GP (1994) Relationships between maternal and developmental toxicity. In: Kimmel CA & Buelke-Sam J ed. Developmental toxicology, 2nd ed. New York, Raven Press, pp 189–212.

Daston GP (1996a) The theoretical and empirical case for *in vitro* developmental toxicity screens, and potential applications. Teratology, **53**: 339–344.

Daston GP (1996b) Other functional abnormalities: methods and data evaluation. In: Hood RD ed. Handbook of developmental toxicology. Boca Raton, Florida, CRC Press, pp 357–381.

Daston GP & Manson JM (1995) Critical periods of exposure and developmental outcome. Inhal Toxicol, **7**: 863–871.

Daston GP, Baines D, Elmore E, Fitzgerald MP, & Sharma S (1995) Evaluation of chick embryo neural retina cell culture as a screen for developmental toxicants. Fundam Appl Toxicol, **26**: 203–210.

Dawson AB (1926) Note on the staining of the skeleton of cleared skeletal specimens with alizarin red S. Stain Technol, **1**: 123–124.

Dawson DA (1991) Additive incidence of developmental malformation for *Xenopus* embryos exposed to a mixture of 10 aliphatic carboxylic acids. Teratology, **44**: 531–546.

Dawson DA & Bantle JA (1987) Development of a reconstituted water medium and a preliminary validation of the frog embryo teratogenesis assay: *Xenopus* (FETAX). J Appl Toxicol, **7**: 237–244.

Dawson EB, Evans DR, & Nosovitch J (1999) Third-trimester amniotic fluid metal levels associated with preeclampsia. Arch Environ Health, **54**: 412–415.

de Cock J, Westveer K, Heederik D, te Velde E, & van Kooij R (1994) Time to pregnancy and occupational exposure to pesticides in fruit growers in the Netherlands. Occup Environ Med, **51**: 693–699.

Diwan BA, Riggs CW, Logsdon D, Haines DC, Olivero OA, Rice JM, Yuspa SH, Poirier MC, & Anderson LM (1999) Multiorgan transplacental and neonatal carcinogenicity of 3′-azido-3′-deoxythymidine in mice. Toxicol Appl Pharmacol, **161**(1): 82–99.

Donovan PJ (1999) Cell sensitivity to transplacental carcinogenesis by *N*-ethyl-*N*-nitrosourea is greatest in early post-implantation development. Mutat Res, **427**(1): 59–63.

Drew R & Miners JO (1984) The effects of buthionine sulphoximine (BSO) on glutathione depletion and xenobiotic biotransformation. Biochem Pharmacol, **33**: 2989–2994.

EC (1990) EEC note for guidance: Good clinical practice for trials on medical products in the European Community. Pharmacol Toxicol, **67**: 361–372.

EC (1994) Commission regulation (EC) No. 1488/94 of 28 June 1994 laying down the principles of the assessment of risks to man and the environment of existing substances in accordance with Council regulation (EEC) No. 793/93. Official Journal of European Communities, L 161. Brussels, European Commission.

EC (1996) Technical guidance document in support of the Commission directive 93/67EEC on risk assessment for new notified substances and Commission regulation 1488/94 EEC on risk assessment for existing chemicals. Brussels, European Commission.

ECETOC (1989) Alternative approaches for the assessment of reproductive toxicity. Brussels, European Centre for Ecotoxicology and Toxicology of Chemicals (Monograph No. 12).

ECETOC (1992) Estimating environmental concentrations of chemicals using fate and exposure models. Brussels, European Centre for Ecotoxicology and Toxicology of Chemicals (Technical Report No. 50).

ECETOC (1996) Environmental estrogens: a compendium of test methods. Brussels, European Centre for Ecotoxicology and Toxicology of Chemicals (ECETOC Document 33).

ECETOC/UNEP (1996) Inventory of critical reviews on chemicals. Brussels, European Centre for Ecotoxicology and Toxicology of Chemicals, and Geneva, United Nations Environment Programme, International Register of Potentially Toxic Chemicals.

Egeland GM, Sweeney MH, Fingerhut MA, Wille KK, Schnorr TM, & Halperin WE (1994) Total serum testosterone and gonadotropins in workers exposed to dioxin. Am J Epidemiol, **139**(3): 272–281.

Eggert-Kruse W, Leinhos G, Gerhard I, Tilgen W, & Runnebaum B (1989) Prognostic value of *in vitro* sperm penetration into hormonally standardized human cervical mucus. Fertil Steril, **51**: 317–323.

Ehrenkranz JRL (1983) Seasonal breeding in humans: birth recordings of the Labrador Eskimos. Fertil Steril, **40**: 485–489.

Eisenberg L (1981) Physiological and psychological aspects of sexual development and function. In: Hamilton DW & Naftolin F ed. Basic reproductive medicine, Vol. 1. Cambridge, Massachusetts, The MIT Press, p 118.

Epidemiology Workshop for the Interagency Regulatory Liaison Group (1981) Guidelines for documentation of epidemiologic studies. Am J Epidemiol, **114**: 609–613.

Erickson GF (1978) Normal ovarian function. Clin Obstet Gynecol, **21**: 31–52.

Evenson DP & Jost LK (1993) Hydroxyurea exposure alters mouse testicular kinetics and sperm chromatin structure. Cell Prolif, **26**: 147–159.

Fabia J & Thuy TD (1974) Occupation of father at time of children dying of malignant disease. Br J Prev Soc Med, **28**: 98–100.

Fantel AG, Greenaway JC, Juchau MR, & Shepard TH (1979) Teratogenic bioactivation of cyclophosphamide *in vitro*. Life Sci, **25**: 67–72.

Faustman EM, Allen BC, Kavlock RJ, & Kimmel CA (1994) Dose–response assessment for developmental toxicity: I. Characterization of data base and determination of NOAELs. Fundam Appl Toxicol, **23**: 478–486.

Ferin MJ (1996) The menstrual cycle: An integrative view. In: Adashi EY, Rock JA, & Rosenwaks Z ed. Reproductive endocrinology, surgery, and technology. Philadelphia, Pennsylvania, Lippincott-Raven Publishers, pp 103–121.

Feychting M, Floderus B, & Ahlbom A (2000) Parental occupational exposure to magnetic fields and childhood cancer (Sweden). Cancer Causes Control **11**: 151–156.

Flint OP (1993) *In vitro* tests for teratogens: Desirable endpoints, test batteries and current status of the micromass teratogen test. Reprod Toxicol, **7**(Suppl 1): 103–111.

Flint OP & Orton TC (1984) An *in vitro* assay for teratogens with cultures of rat embryo midbrain and limb cells. Toxicol Appl Pharmacol, **76**: 383–395.

Foster WG (1992) Reproductive toxicity of chronic lead exposure in the female cynomolgus monkey. Reprod Toxicol, **6**: 123–131.

Foster WG, McMahon A, YoungLai EV, Jarrell JF, & Lecavalier P (1995) Alterations in circulating ovarian steroids in hexachlorobenzene exposed monkeys. Reprod Toxicol, **9**: 541–548.

Foster W, Chan S, Platt L, & Hughes C (2000) Detection of endocrine disrupting chemicals in samples of second trimester human amniotic fluid. J Clin Endocrinol Metab, **85**: 2954–2957.

Francis EZ, Kimmel CA, & Rees DC (1990) Workshop on the qualitative and quantitative comparability of human and animal developmental neurotoxicity: summary and implications. Neurotoxicol Teratol, **12**(3): 285–292.

Garcia AM, Benavides FG, Fletcher T, & Orts E (1998) Paternal exposure to pesticides and congenital malformations. Scand J Work Environ Health, **24**: 473–480.

Gardner MJ, Snee MP, Hall AJ, Powell CA, Downes S, & Terrell JD (1990) Results of case–control study of leukemia and lymphoma among young people near Sellafield nuclear plant in West Cumbria. Br Med J, **300**(6722): 423–429.

Generoso WM, Rutledge JC, Cain KT, Hughes LA, & Braden PW (1987) Exposure of female mice to ethylene oxide within hours of mating leads to fetal malformation and death. Mutat Res, **176**: 269–274.

Generoso WM, Rutledge JC, Cain KT, Hughes LA, & Downing DJ (1988) Mutagen-induced fetal anomalies and death following treatment of females within hours after mating. Mutat Res, **199**: 175–181.

Genschow E, Scholz G, Brown N, Piersma A, Brady M, Clemann N, Huuskonen H, Paillard F, Bremer S, Becker K, & Spielmann H (2000) Development of prediction models for three *in vitro* embryotoxicity tests in an ECVAM validation study. In Vitro Mol Toxicol, **13**(1): 51–66.

Gillman J, Gilbert C, Gillman T, & Spence I (1948) A preliminary report on hydrocephalus, spina bifida and other anomalies in the rat produced by trypan blue. S Afr J Med Sci, **13**: 47–90.

Goebelsmann U (1986) The menstrual cycle. In: Mishell DR & Davajan V ed. Fertility, contraception and reproductive endocrinology, 2nd ed. Oradell, New Jersey, Medical Economics, pp 71–73.

Gold EB & Sever LE (1994) Childhood cancers associated with parental occupational exposures. Occup Med, **9**: 495–539.

Goldstein A, Aronow L, & Kalman SM (1968) The absorption, distribution and elimination of drugs — passage of drugs across the placenta. In: Goldstein A, Aronow L, & Kalman SM ed. Principles of drug action: the basis of pharmacology. New York, Harper and Row, p 179.

Gore-Langton RE & Armstrong DT (1994) Follicular steroidogenesis and its control. In: Knobil RE & Neil JD ed. The physiology of reproduction, 2nd ed. New York, Raven Press, pp 571–627.

Gospodarowicz D (1989) Fibroblast growth factor. Crit Rev Oncol, **1**: 1–26.

Gourbin C & Masuy-Strobant G (1995) Registration of vital data: are live births and stillbirths comparable all over Europe? Bull WHO, **73**: 449–460.

Grant LD (1976) Research strategies for behavioral teratology studies. Environ Health Perspect, **18**: 85–94.

Gray A, Feldman HA, McKinlay JB, & Longcope C (1991) Age, disease, and changing sex hormone levels in middle-aged men: Results of the Massachusetts male aging study. J Clin Endocrinol Metab, **73**: 1016–1025.

Gray LE, Ostby J, Sigmon R, Ferrell J, Linder R, Cooper R, Goldman J, & Laskey J (1988) The development of a protocol to assess reproductive effects of toxicants in the rat. Reprod Toxicol, **2**: 281–287.

Greenberg JH (1982) Detection of teratogens by differentiating embryonic neural crest cells in culture; evaluation as a screening system. Teratog Carcinog Mutagen, **2**: 319–323.

Greenwald GS (1987) Possible animal models of follicular development relevant to reproductive toxicology. Reprod Toxicol, **1**: 55–59.

Guthrie HD, Grimes RW, & Hammond JM (1995) Changes in insulin-like growth factor binding protein-1 and -3 in follicular fluid during atresia of follicles grown after ovulation in pigs. J Reprod Fertil, **104**: 225–230.

Handelsman DJ, Wishart S, & Conway AJ (2000) Oestradiol enhances testosterone-induced suppression of human spermatogenesis. Hum Reprod, **15**(3): 672–679.

Harry GJ ed. (1994) Developmental toxicology. Boca Raton, Florida, CRC Press, p 177.

Health Canada (1994) Human health risk assessment for Priority Substances. Ottawa, Ontario, Health Canada, Environmental Health Directorate, Canada Communication Group — Publishing (Publication No. En40-215/41E).

Heindel JJ (1998) Oocyte quantitation and ovarian histology. In: Daston G & Kimmel C ed. An evaluation of reproductive endpoints for human health risk assessment. Washington, DC, ILSI Press, pp 57–74.

Heindel JJ & Chapin RE ed. (1993) Methods in toxicology 3b: Female reproductive toxicology. San Diego, California, Academic Press.

Hemminki K & Vineis P (1985) Extrapolation of the evidence on teratogenicity of chemicals between humans and experimental animals: Chemicals other than drugs. Teratog Carcinog Mutagen, **5**: 251–318.

Hemminki K, Mutanen P, Luoma K, & Saloniemi I (1980) Congenital malformations by the parental occupation in Finland. Int Arch Occup Environ Health, **46**: 93–98.

Hemminki K, Saloniemi I, & Salonen T (1981) Childhood cancer and paternal occupation in Finland. J Epidemiol Community Health, **35**: 11–15.

Herbst AL, Ulfelder H, & Poskanzer DC (1971) Adenocarcinoma of the vagina. Association of maternal stilbestrol therapy with tumour appearance in young women. N Engl J Med, **284**: 878–881.

Hertel RF (1996) Outline on risk assessment of existing substances in the European Union. Environ Toxicol Pharmacol, **2**: 93–96.

Hess RA (1990) Quantitative and qualitative characteristics of the stages and transitions in the cycle of the rat seminiferous epithelium: light microscopic observations of perfusion-fixed and plastic-embedded testes. Biol Reprod, **43**: 525–542.

Hess RA & Moore BJ (1993) Histological methods for evaluation of the testis. In: Chapin RE & Heindel JJ ed. Methods in toxicology 3a: Male reproductive toxicology. San Diego, California, Academic Press, pp 52–85.

Hill RB (1965) The environment and disease: association or causation. Proc R Soc Med, **58**: 295–300.

Holson RR, Paule MG, & Scalzo FM ed. (1990) Methods in behavioral toxicology and teratology. Neurotoxicol Teratol, **12**(5).

Hubel CA (1999) Oxidative stress in the pathogenesis of preeclampsia. Proc Soc Exp Biol Med **222**: 222–235.

Hughes EW & Palmer AK (1980) An assessment of preweaning development and behaviour in safety evaluation studies. Abstracts of the Annual Meeting of the Experimental Teratology Society, Munster.

Hwang SJ, Beaty TH, Panny SR, Street NA, Joseph JM, Gordon S, McIntosh I, & Francomano CA (1995) Association study of transforming growth factor alpha (TGF)–environment interaction in a population-based sample of infants with birth defects. Am J Epidemiol, **141**: 629–636.

IARC (1980) Long-term and short-term screening assays for carcinogens: a critical appraisal. Lyon, International Agency for Research on Cancer, 426 pp (IARC Monographs on the Evaluation of the Carcinogenic Risk of Chemicals to Humans, Suppl 2).

ICH (1993) ICH Harmonised Tripartite Guideline: Detection of toxicity to reproduction for medicinal products. International Conference on Harmonisation of Technical Requirements for Registration of Pharmaceuticals for Human Use.

ILSI (1999) An evaluation and interpretation of reproductive endpoints for human health risk assessment. Washington, DC, International Life Sciences Institute Press.

Imagawa W, Yang J, Guzman R, & Nandi S (1994) Control of mammary gland development. In: Knobil E & Neill JD ed. The physiology of reproduction. New York, Raven Press, pp 1033–1063.

Inouye M (1976) Differential staining of cartilage and bone in mouse skeleton by alcian blue and alizarin red S. Congenital Anomalies, **16**: 171–173.

International Clearing House (1991) Congenital malformations worldwide. A report from the International Clearing House for Birth Defects Monitoring Systems. Amsterdam, Elsevier.

IPCS (1984) Environmental health criteria 30: Principles for evaluating health risks to progeny associated with exposure to chemicals during pregnancy. Geneva, World Health Organization, International Programme on Chemical Safety.

IPCS (1986a) Environmental health criteria 59: Principles for evaluating health risks from chemicals during infancy and early childhood: The need for a special approach. Geneva, World Health Organization, International Programme on Chemical Safety.

IPCS (1986b) Environmental health criteria 60: Principles and methods for the assessment of neurotoxicity associated with exposure to chemicals. Geneva, World Health Organization, International Programme on Chemical Safety.

IPCS (1986c) Environmental health criteria 57: Principles of toxicokinetic studies. Geneva, World Health Organization, International Programme on Chemical Safety.

IPCS (1987) Environmental health criteria 70: Principles for the safety assessment of food additives and contaminants in food. Geneva, World Health Organization, International Programme on Chemical Safety.

IPCS (1992) Environmental health criteria 144: Principles for evaluating the effects of chemicals on the aged population. Geneva, World Health Organization, International Programme on Chemical Safety.

IPCS (1994) Environmental health criteria 170: Assessing human health risks to chemicals: derivation of guidance values for health-based exposure limits. Geneva, World Health Organization, International Programme on Chemical Safety.

IPCS (1995) International Programme on Chemical Safety/Organisation for Economic Co-operation and Development Workshop on the Harmonization of Risk Assessment for Reproductive and Development Toxicity, 17–21 October 1994. Carshalton, Surrey, United Kingdom, BIBRA International (IPCS/95.25).

IPCS (1996) Environmental health criteria 180: Principles and methods for the assessment of immunotoxicity associated with exposures to chemicals. Geneva, World Health Organization, International Programme on Chemical Safety.

IPCS (1999) Environmental health criteria 210: Principles for the assessment of risks to human health from exposure to chemicals. Geneva, World Health Organization, International Programme on Chemical Safety.

IPCS (2001a) Environmental health criteria 223: Neurotoxicity risk assessment for human health: Principles and approaches. Geneva, World Health Organization, International Programme on Chemical Safety.

IPCS (2001b) Guidance document for the use of data in development of chemical-specific adjustment factors (CSAFs) for interspecies differences and human variability in dose/concentration–response assessment (draft). Prepared as part of the IPCS project on the Harmonization of Approaches to the Assessment of Risk from Exposure. Geneva, World Health Organization, International Programme on Chemical Safety.

Irvine S, Cawood E, Richardson D, MacDonald E, & Aitken J (1996) Evidence of deteriorating semen quality in the United Kingdom: birth cohort study in 577 men in Scotland over 11 years. Br Med J, **312**: 467–471.

IUPAC (1998) Natural and anthropogenic environmental oestrogens. J Int Union Pure Appl Chem, **70**: 1617–1865.

Ivankovic S & Druckrey H (1968) Carcinogenesis in the progeny after exposure of pregnant animals. Food Cosmet Toxicol, **6**(5): 584–585.

Jacobson JL & Jacobson SW (1996) Intellectual impairment in children exposed to polychlorinated biphenyls *in utero*. N Engl J Med, **335**: 783–789.

Janecki A & Steinberger A (1986) Polarized Sertoli cell functions in a new two-compartment culture system. J Androl, **7**(1): 69–71.

Jankowski-Hennig MA, Clegg MS, Daston GP, Rogers JM, & Keen CL (2000) Zinc-deficient rat embryos have increased caspase 3-like activity and apoptosis. Biochem Biophys Res Commun, **271**(1): 250–256.

Jansen HT, Cooke PS, Porcelli J, Liu T, & Hansen LG (1993) Estrogenic and antiestrogenic actions of PCBs in the female rat. *In vitro* and *in vivo* studies. Reprod Toxicol, **7**: 237–248.

Jarrell JF, Villeneuve D, Franklin C, Bartlett S, Wrixon W, Kohut J, & Zouves CG (1993) Contamination of human ovarian follicular fluid and serum by chlorinated organic compounds in three Canadian cities. Can Med Assoc J, **148**: 1321–1327.

Jarrell JF, Gocmen A, Foster WG, Brant R, Chan S, & Sevcik M (1996) Evaluation of reproductive outcomes in women inadvertently exposed to hexachlorobenzene in southeastern Turkey in the 1950's. Reprod Toxicol, **12**: 469–476.

Jelinek R & Peterka M (1981) Morphogenetic systems and *in vitro* techniques in teratology. In: Neubert D & Merker H-J ed. Culture techniques. Applicability for studies on prenatal differentiation and toxicity. Berlin, New York, Walter de Gruyter Publishers, pp 553–557.

Joffe M (1985) Biases in research on reproductive and women's work. Int J Epidemiol, **14**: 118–123.

Joffe M, Bisanti L, Apostoli P, Shah N, Kiss P, Dale A, Roeleveld N, Lindbohm ML, Sallmen M, & Bonde JP (1999) Time to pregnancy and occupational lead exposure. Asclepios. Scand J Work Environ Health, **25**(1): 64–65.

Johnson EM, Newman LM, Gabel BEG, Boerner TF, & Dansky LA (1988) An analysis of the hydra assay's applicability and reliability as a developmental toxicity prescreen. J Am Coll Toxicol, **7**: 111–126.

Johnson L, Petty CS, & Neaves WB (1983) Further quantification of human spermatogenesis: Germ cell loss during postprophase of meiosis and its relationship to daily sperm production. Biol Reprod, **29**: 207.

Jorgensen N, Auger J, Giwercman A, Irvine DS, Jensen TK, Jouannet P, Keiding N, Le Bon C, MacDonald E, Pekuri AM, Scheike T, Simonsen M, Suominen M, Suominen J, & Skakkebaaek NE (1997) Semen analysis performed by different laboratory teams: an intervention study. Int J Androl, **20**: 201–208.

Jouannet P, Czyglik F, David G, Mayaux MJ, Spira A, Moscato ML, & Schwartz D (1981) Study of a group of 484 fertile men. Part 1. Distribution of semen characteristics. Int J Androl, **4**: 440–449.

Juchau MR (1980) Drug biotransformation in the placenta. Pharmacol Ther, **8**: 501–524.

Juul S, Karmmaus W, & Olsen J (1999) Regional differences in waiting time to pregnancy: pregnancy-based surveys from Denmark, France, Germany, Italy and Sweden. The European Infertility and Subfecundity Study Group. Hum Reprod, **14**: 1250–1254.

Kangasniemi M, Veromaa T, Kulmala J, Parvinen M, & Toppari J (1990) DNA flow cytometry of defined stages of rat seminiferous epithelium: effects of 3 Gy of high energy x-irradiation. J Androl, **11**: 312–317.

Katoh M, Cacheiro NLA, Cornett CV, Cain KT, Rutledge JC, & Generoso WM (1989) Fetal anomalies produced subsequent to treatment of zygotes with ethylene oxide or ethyl methanesulfonate are not likely due to the unusual genetic causes. Mutat Res, **210**: 337–344.

Kavlock RJ & Daston GP (1997) Drug toxicity in embryonic development, Vol. 1 and 2. Heidelberg, Springer Verlag.

Kavlock RJ, Allen BC, Kimmel CA, & Faustman EM (1995) Dose–response assessment for developmental toxicity: IV. Benchmark doses for fetal weight changes. Fundam Appl Toxicol, **26**: 211–222.

Kavlock RJ, Daston GP, DeRosa C, Fenner-Crisp P, Gray LE, Kaaten S, Lucier G, Luster M, Mac M, Maczka C, Miller R, Moore J, Rolland R, Scott G, Sheehan DM, Sinks T, & Tilson HA (1996) Research needs for assessment of health and environmental effects of endocrine disruptors: A report of the US EPA sponsored workshop. Environ Health Perspect, **104**: 715–740.

Keen CL, Peters JM, & Hurley LS (1989) The effect of valproic acid on ^{65}Zn distribution in the pregnant rat. J Nutr, **119**: 607–611.

Khera KS (1984) Adverse effects in humans and animals of prenatal exposure to selected therapeutic drugs and estimation of embryo-fetal sensitivity of animals for human risk assessment: A review. In: Kalter H ed. Issues and reviews in teratology, Vol. 2. New York, Plenum Press, pp 399–508.

Khoury MJ & Holtzman NA (1987) On the ability of birth defects monitoring to detect new teratogens. Am J Epidemiol, **126**: 136–143.

Kimmel CA (1990) Quantitative approaches to human risk assessment for noncancer health effects. Neurotoxicology, **11**: 189–198.

Kimmel CA & Buelke-Sam J ed. (1994) Developmental toxicology, 2nd ed. New York, Raven Press.

Kimmel CA & Gaylor DW (1988) Issues in qualitative and quantitative risk analysis for developmental toxicology. J Risk Anal, **8**: 15–20.

Kimmel CA & Kimmel GL (1994) Risk assessment for developmental toxicity. In: Kimmel CA & Buelke-Sam J ed. Developmental toxicology, 2nd ed. New York, Raven Press, pp 429–453.

Kimmel CA & Kimmel GL (1996) Principles of developmental toxicology risk assessment. In: Hood RD ed. Handbook of developmental toxicology. Boca Raton, Florida, CRC Press, pp 667–693.

Kimmel CA, Holson JF, Hogue CJ, & Carlo GL (1984) Reliability of experimental studies for predicting hazards to human development. Jefferson, Arkansas, National Center for Toxicological Research (NCTR Technical Report for Experimental Studies No. 6015).

Kimmel CA, Kimmel GL, & Frankos V ed. (1986) Interagency Regulatory Liaison Group workshop on reproductive toxicity risk assessment. Environ Health Perspect, **66**: 193–221.

Kimmel CA, Rees DC, & Francis EZ ed. (1990) Proceedings of the workshop on the qualitative and quantitative comparability of human and animal developmental neurotoxicity. Neurotoxicol Teratol, **12**: 173–292.

Kimmel GL & Kochhar DM (1990) *In vitro* methods in developmental toxicology: use in defining mechanisms and risk parameters. Boca Raton, Florida, CRC Press.

Kimmel GL, Clegg ED, & Crisp TM (1995) Reproductive toxicity testing: a risk assessment perspective. In: Witorsch RJ ed. Reproductive toxicology. New York, Raven Press, pp 75–98.

Kitchin KT, Sanyal MK, & Schmid BP (1981) A coupled microsomal activating/embryo culture system: Toxicity of reduced β-nicotinamide adenine dinucleotide phosphate (NADPH). Biochem Pharmacol, **30**: 985–992.

Klaassen CD, Amdur MO, & Doull J ed. (1996) Casarett and Doull's toxicology: The basic science of poisons, 5th ed. New York, McGraw-Hill.

Klein KO, Baron J, Colli MJ, McDonnell DP, & Cutler GBJ (1994) Estrogen levels in childhood determined by an ultrasensitive recombinant cell bioassay. J Clin Invest, **94**: 2475–2480.

Kleinbaum DG, Kupper LL, & Morgenstern H (1982) Epidemiologic research: Principles and quantitative methods. London, Lifetime Learning Publications.

Knecht M, Feng P, & Catt KJ (1989) Transforming growth factor-beta: Autocrine, paracrine, and endocrine effects in ovarian cells. Semin Reprod Endocrinol, **7**: 20–26.

Knobil E (1980) The neuroendocrine control of the menstrual cycle. Recent Prog Horm Res, **36**: 53–88.

Knobil E & Neill JD ed. (1994) The physiology of reproduction, 2nd ed. 2 vols. New York, Raven Press.

Knudsen I, Hansen EV, Meyer AO, & Poulsen E (1977) A proposed method for the simultaneous detection of germ-cell mutations leading to foetal death (dominant lethality) and of malformations (male teratogenicity) in mammals. Mutat Res, **478**: 267–270.

Koos RD (1989) Potential relevance of angiogenic factors to ovarian physiology. Semin Reprod Endocrinol, **7**: 29–33.

Kramer MS (1987) Determinants of low birth weight: methodological assessment and meta-analysis. Bull WHO, **65**: 663–737.

Krzyzanowski M (2000) Evaluation and use of epidemiological evidence for environmental health risk assessment: WHO guideline document. Environ Health Perspect, **108**(10): 997–1002.

Kwa SL & Fine LJ (1980) The association between parental occupation and childhood malignancy. J Occup Med, **22**: 792–794.

LaKind JS, Berlin CM, & Naiman DQ (2001) Infant exposure to chemicals in breast milk in the United States: what we need to learn from a breast monitoring program. Environ Health Perspect, **109**(1): 75–88.

Lamb JC (1985) Reproductive toxicity testing: evaluating and developing new testing systems. J Am Coll Toxicol, **4**: 163–171.

Landrigan PJ, Weiss B, Goldman LR, Carpenter DO, & Suk WA ed. (2000) The developing brain and the environment. Environ Health Perspect, 108(Suppl 3): 373–595.

Larsen SB, Spano M, Giwercman A, & Bonde JP (1999) Semen quality and sex hormones among organic and traditional Danish farmers. ASCLEPIOS Study Group. Occup Environ Med, 56: 139–144.

Lau C, Andersen ME, Crawford-Brown DJ, Kavlock RJ, Kimmel CA, Knudsen TB, Muneoka K, Rogers JM, Setzer RW, Smith G, & Tyl R (2000) Evaluation of biologically based dose–response modeling for developmental toxicity: A workshop report. Regul Toxicol Pharmacol, 31(2 Pt 1): 190–199.

Laumon B, Martin JL, Collet P, Bertucat I, Verney MP, & Robert E (1996) Exposure to organic solvents during pregnancy and oral clefts: a case–control study. Reprod Toxicol, 10(1): 15–19 [published erratum appears in Reprod Toxicol 1996, 10(3): vi].

LeFevre J & McClintock MK (1988) Reproductive senescence in female rats: A longitudinal study of individual differences in estrous cycles and behaviour. Biol Reprod, 38: 780–789.

Lemasters GK (1993) Epidemiology methods to assess occupational exposures and pregnancy outcomes. Semin Perinatol, 17(1): 18–27.

Lemasters GK & Pinney SM (1989) Employment status as a confounder when assessing occupational exposures and spontaneous abortion. J Clin Epidemiol, 42: 975–981.

Leridon H (1977) Human fertility. The basic components. Chicago, Illinois, University of Chicago Press.

Lightman A, Palumno A, DeCherney AH, & Naftolin F (1989) The ovarian renin–angiotensin system. Semin Reprod Endocrinol, 7: 79–84.

Lin S, Hwang SA, Marshall EG, Stone R, & Chen J (1996) Fertility rates among lead workers and professional bus drivers: a comparative study. Ann Epidemiol, 6: 201–208.

Lin T, Blaisdell J, & Haskell JF (1987) Transforming growth factor-beta inhibits Leydig cell steroidogenesis in primary culture. Biochem Biophys Res Commun, 146: 387–394.

Lindbohm ML (1999) Women's reproductive health: some recent developments in occupational epidemiology. Am J Ind Med, 36: 18–24.

Lindbohm ML, Hemminki K, Bonhomme MG, Anttila A, Rantala K, Keikkila P, & Rosenberg MJ (1991) Effects of paternal occupational exposure on spontaneous abortions. Am J Public Health, 81: 1029–1033.

Lindenau A & Fischer B (1996) Embryotoxicity of polychlorinated biphenyls (PCBs) for preimplantation embryos. Reprod Toxicol, 10: 227–230.

Lindsey S & Wilkinson MF (1996) Homeobox genes and male reproductive development. J Assist Reprod Genet, 13: 182–192.

Little RE, Monaghan SC, Gladen BC, Shkryak-Nyzhnyk ZA, & Wilcox AJ (1999) Outcomes of 17,137 pregnancies in 2 urban areas of Ukraine. Am J Public Health, 89: 1832–1836.

Lorente C, Cordier S, Bergeret A, De Walle HE, Goujard J, Ayme S, Knill-Jones R, Calzolari E, & Bianchi F (2000) Maternal occupational risk factors for oral clefts. Occupational Exposure and Congenital Malformation Working Group. Scand J Work Environ Health, **26**: 137–145.

Lorenz J, Glatt HR, Fleischmann R, Ferlinz R, & Oesch F (1984) Drug metabolism in man and in relationship to that in three rodent species: Monooxygenase, epoxide hydrolase and glutathione S-transferase activities in subcellular fractions of lung and liver. Biochem Med, **32**: 43–56.

Lucky AW, Schreiber JR, Hillier SG, Schulman JD, & Ross GT (1977) Progesterone production by cultured preantral rat granulosa cells; stimulation by androgens. Endocrinology, **100**: 128–133.

Mackerprang M, Hay S, & Lunde AS (1972) Completeness and accuracy of reporting of malformations on birth certificates. HSMHA Health Rep, **84**: 43–49.

Maier DB, Newbold RR, & McLachlan JA (1985) Prenatal diethylstilbestrol exposure alters murine uterine responses to prepubertal estrogen stimulation. Endocrinology, **116**: 1878–1886.

Mark M, Rijli FM, & Chambon P (1997) Homeobox genes in embryogenesis and pathogenesis. Pediatr Res, **42**: 421–429.

Matsumoto AM (1996) Spermatogenesis. In: Adashi EY, Rock JA, & Rosenwaks Z ed. Reproductive endocrinology, surgery, and technology. Philadelphia, Pennsylvania, Lippincott-Raven Publishers, pp 359–384.

Mattison DR & Thomford PJ (1989) The mechanisms of action of reproductive toxicants. Toxicol Pathol, **17**: 364–376.

May JV & Schomberg DW (1989) The potential of epidermal growth factor and transforming growth factor-alpha to ovarian physiology. Semin Reprod Endocrinol, **7**: 1–6.

McDonald AD, McDonald JC, Armstrong B, Cherry NM, Nolin AD, & Robert D (1989) Father's occupation and pregnancy outcome. Br J Ind Med, **46**: 329–333.

McGregor AJ & Mason HJ (1990) Chronic occupational lead exposure and testicular endocrine function. Hum Exp Toxicol **9**(6): 371–376.

McGregor AJ & Mason HJ (1991) Occupational mercury vapour exposure and testicular, pituitary and thyroid endocrine function. Hum Exp Toxicol **10**(3): 199–203.

McLachlan JA & Newbold R (1989) End points for assessing reproductive toxicology in the female. In: Working PK ed. Toxicology of the male and female reproductive systems. New York, Hemisphere Publishing, pp 173–178.

Meistrich ML (1982) Quantitative correlation between testicular stem cell survival, sperm production, and fertility in the mouse after treatment with different cytotoxic agents. J Androl, **3**: 58–68.

Meistrich ML & Brown CC (1983) Estimation of the increased risk of human infertility from alterations in semen characteristics. Fertil Steril, **40**: 220–230.

Mirkes PE (1996) Prospects for the development of validated screening tests that measure developmental toxicity potential: View of one skeptic. Teratology, **53**: 334–338.

Mirkin BL & Singh S (1976) Placental transfer of pharmacologically active molecules. In: Mirkin BL ed. Perinatal pharmacology and therapeutics. New York, Academic Press, pp 1–69.

Moller H & Skakkebaek NE (1997) Testicular cancer and cryptorchidism in relation to prenatal factors: case–control studies in Denmark. Cancer Causes Control, 8: 904–912.

Moolgavkar SH (1995) When and how to combine results from multiple epidemiological studies in risk assessment. In: Graham JD ed. The role of epidemiology in regulatory risk assessment. Amsterdam, Elsevier Press.

Moore JA (1995) An assessment of lithium using the IEHR evaluative process for assessing human development and reproductive toxicity of agents. IEHR Expert Scientific Committee. Reprod Toxicol, 9: 175–210.

Moore JA (1997) An assessment of boric acid and borax using the IEHR evaluative process for assessing human developmental and reproductive toxicity of agents. Expert Scientific Committee. Reprod Toxicol, 11: 123–160.

Moore JA, Daston GP, Faustman E, Golub MS, Hart WL, Hughes C Jr, Kimmel CA, Lamb JC IV, Schwetz BA, & Scialli AR (1995) An evaluation process for assessing human reproductive and developmental toxicity of agents. Reprod Toxicol, 9: 61–95.

Moore KL ed. (1988) The developing human. Philadelphia, Pennsylvania, W.B. Saunders.

Moore ML, Michielutte R, Meis PJ, Ernest JM, Wells HB, & Buescher PA (1994) Etiology of low-birthweight birth: A population-based study. Prev Med, 23: 793–799.

Morrissey RE, Lamb JC, Schwetz BA, Teague JL, & Morris RW (1988a) Association of sperm, vaginal cytology, and reproductive organ weight data with results of continuous breeding reproduction studies in Swiss (CD-1) mice. Fundam Appl Toxicol, 11: 359–371.

Morrissey RE, Schwetz BA, Lamb JC, Ross MD, Teague JL, & Morris RW (1988b) Evaluation of rodent sperm, vaginal cytology, and reproductive organ weight data from National Toxicology Program 13 week studies. Fundam Appl Toxicol, 11: 343–358.

Morrissey RE, Lamb JC, Morris RW, Chapin RE, Gulati DK, & Heindel JJ (1989) Results and evaluations of 48 continuous breeding reproduction studies conducted in mice. Fundam Appl Toxicol, 13: 747–777.

Moser VC & MacPhail RC (1989) Neurobehavioural effect of triadimefon, a triazole fungicide, in male and female rats. Neurotoxicol Teratol, 11(3): 285–293.

Mul T, Mongelli M, & Gardosi J (1996) A comparative analysis of second-trimester ultrasound dating formulae in pregnancies conceived with artificial reproductive techniques. Ultrasound Obstet Gynecol, 8(6): 397–402.

Müller WF, Hobson W, Fuller GB, Knauf W, Coulston F, & Korte F (1978) Endocrine effects of chlorinated hydrocarbons in rhesus monkeys. Ecotoxicol Environ Saf, 2: 161–172.

Mummery CL, Slager HG, Van Inzen W, Freund E, & van den Eijnden-van Raaij AJM (1993) Regulation of growth and differentiation in early development: Of mice and models. Reprod Toxicol, 7(Suppl 1): 145–154.

Nakai M, Moore BJ, & Hess RA (1993) Epithelial reorganization and irregular growth following carbendazim-induced injury of the efferent ductules of the rat testis. Anat Rec, 235: 51–60.

Nau H (1985) Teratogenic valproic acid concentrations: infusion by implanted minipumps vs. conventional injection regimen in the mouse. Toxicol Appl Pharmacol, **80**: 243–250.

Nau H (1987) Species differences in pharmacokinetics, drug metabolism and teratogenesis. In: Nau H & Scott WJ Jr ed. Pharmacokinetics in teratogenesis, Vol. 1. Boca Raton, Florida, CRC Press, pp 81–106.

Nau H & Liddiard C (1978) Placental transfer of drugs during early human pregnancy. In: Neubert D, Merker H-J, Nau H, & Langman J ed. Role of pharmacokinetics in prenatal and perinatal toxicology. Stuttgart, Georg Thieme, pp 465–481.

Nau H & Scott WJ Jr ed. (1987) Pharmacokinetics in teratogenesis. 2 vols. Boca Raton, Florida, CRC Press.

Nebert DW, Dalton TP, Stuart GW, & Carvan MJ III (2000) "Gene-swap knock-in" cassette in mice to study allelic differences in human genes. Ann NY Acad Sci, **919**: 148–170.

Neubert D (1980) Teratogenicity: Any relationship to carcinogenicity? In: Montesano R, Bartsch H, Tomatis L, & Davis W ed. Molecular and cellular aspects of carcinogen screening tests. Lyon, International Agency for Research on Cancer (IARC Scientific Publications No. 27).

Neubert D (1982) The use of culture techniques in studies on prenatal toxicity. Pharm Ther, **18**: 397–434.

New DAT (1978) Whole embryo culture and the study of mammalian embryos during organogenesis. Biol Rev, **53**: 81–122.

Newbold RR, Hanson RB, Jefferson WN, Bullick BC, Haseman J, & McLachlan JA (1998) Increased tumors but uncompromised fertility in the female descendants of mice exposed developmentally to diethylstilbestrol. Carcinogenesis, **19**(9): 1655–1663.

Newbold RR, Hanson RB, Jefferson WN, Bullick BC, Haseman J, & McLachlan JA (2000) Proliferative lesions and reproductive tract tumors in male descendants of mice exposed developmentally to diethylstilbestrol. Carcinogenesis, **21**(7): 1355–1363.

Newman LM, Johnson EM, & Staples RE (1993) Assessment of the effectiveness of animal developmental toxicity testing for human safety. Reprod Toxicol, **7**: 359–390.

Niederreither K, Ward SJ, Dolle P, & Chambon P (1996) Morphological and molecular characterization of retinoic acid-induced limb duplications in mice. Dev Biol, **176**(2): 185–198.

Nisbet ICT & Karch NJ (1983) Chemical hazards to human reproduction. Park Ridge, New Jersey, Noyes Data Corporation.

Nomura T (1982) Parental exposure to X-rays and chemicals induces heritable tumours and anomalies in mice. Nature, **296**: 575–577.

Nonaka K, Miura T, & Peter K (1994) Recent fertility decline in Dariusleut Hutterites: an extension of Eaton and Mayer's Hutterite fertility study. Hum Biol, **66**: 411–420.

Nothdurft H & Sterz H (1977) Routine radiography of the skeletons of 31-day-old rabbit fetuses. In: Neubert D, Merker H-J, & Kwasigroch TE ed. Methods in prenatal toxicology. Stuttgart, Georg Thieme, pp 155–164.

OECD (1981a) Test Guideline 414: Teratogenicity. Paris, Organisation for Economic Co-operation and Development.

OECD (1981b) Test Guideline 453: Combined chronic toxicity/carcinogenicity studies. Paris, Organisation for Economic Co-operation and Development.

OECD (1983a) Test Guideline 415: One generation reproduction toxicity. Paris, Organisation for Economic Co-operation and Development.

OECD (1983b) Test Guideline 416: Two generation reproduction toxicity. Paris, Organisation for Economic Co-operation and Development.

OECD (1989) Compendium of environmental exposure assessment methods for chemicals. Paris, Organisation for Economic Co-operation and Development (Environmental Monograph No. 27).

OECD (1995) Test Guideline 421: Reproduction/developmental toxicity. Paris, Organisation for Economic Co-operation and Development.

OECD (1996a) Guidelines for pesticides and industrial chemicals. Paris, Organisation for Economic Co-operation and Development.

OECD (1996b) Test Guideline 422: Combined repeated dose toxicity with reproduction/developmental toxicity screening. Paris, Organisation for Economic Co-operation and Development.

OECD (1998a) Report of the First Meeting of the OECD Endocrine Disruptor Testing and Assessment (EDTA) Working Group, 10–11 March 1998. Paris, Organisation for Economic Co-operation and Development (ENV/MC/CHEM/RA(98)5).

OECD (1998b) Report of the Second Meeting of the Joint National Coordinators Meeting/Risk Assessment Advisory Board (NCM/RAAB) Working Group on Endocrine Disruptor Testing and Assessment (EDTA Task Force), 12–13 November 1998. Paris, Organisation for Economic Co-operation and Development.

OECD (1999a) Report of OECD Task Force on Endocrine Disruptor Testing and Assessment. Paris, Organisation for Economic Co-operation and Development.

OECD (1999b) Final record: First Meeting of the OECD Validation Management Committee for the Screening and Testing of Endocrine Disrupting Substances — Mammalian Effects, Tokyo, Japan, 8–10 February 1999. Paris, Organisation for Economic Co-operation and Development.

OECD (1999c) Test Guideline 426: Prenatal developmental neurotoxicity study (draft). Paris, Organisation for Economic Co-operation and Development.

OECD (2001a) Test Guideline 414: Prenatal developmental toxicity. Paris, Organisation for Economic Co-operation and Development.

OECD (2001b) Test Guideline 416: Two generation reproduction toxicity. Paris, Organisation for Economic Co-operation and Development.

OECD/IPCS (2001) Project on the harmonization of chemical hazard/risk assessment terminology: Critical analysis of survey results. Organisation for Economic Co-operation and Development and World Health Organization, International Programme on Chemical Safety (in press).

Oglesby LA, Ebron MT, Beyer BE, Carver BD, & Kavlock RJ (1986) Cocultures of rat embryos and hepatocytes: *In vitro* detection of a proteratogen. Teratog Carcinog Mutagen, **6**: 129–138.

Olsson PE, Borg B, Brunström B, Håkansson H, & Klasson-Wheler E (1998) Endocrine-disrupting substances — Impairment of reproduction. Stockholm, Swedish Environmental Protection Agency Customer Services.

Palmer AK (1977) Incidence of sporadic malformations, anomalies and variations in random bred laboratory animals. In: Neubert D, Merker H-J, & Kwasigroch TE ed. Methods in prenatal toxicology. Stuttgart, Georg Thieme, pp 52–71.

Papier CM (1985) Parental occupation and congenital malformations in a series of 35,000 births in Israel. Prog Clin Biol Res, **163**: 291–294.

Parker KI, Ikeda Y, & Luo X (1996) The roles of steroidogenic factor-1 in reproductive function. Steroids, **61**: 161–165.

Pellegrini M, Pantano S, Lucchini F, Fumi M, & Forabosco A (1997) Emx2 developmental expression in the primordia of the reproductive and excretory systems. Anal Embryol (Berl), **196**: 427–433.

Peltoketo H, Nokelainen P, Paio YS, Vihko R, & Vihko P (1999) Two 17β-hydroxysteroid dehydrogenases (17HSDs) of estriadol biosynthesis 17HSD type 1 and type 7. J Steroid Biochem Mol Biol, **69**(1–6): 431–439.

Peters JM, Preston-Martin S, & Yu MC (1981) Brain tumors in children and occupational exposure of the parents. Science, **213**: 235–237.

Piersma AH, Verhoef A, & Peters PWJ (1991) Effects of low sodium concentrations on the development of postimplantation rat embryos in culture and on their sensitivity to anticonvulsants. Toxicol In Vitro, **1**: 71–75.

Piersma AH, Attenon P, Bechter R, Govers MJAP, Krafft N, Schmid BP, Stadler J, Verhoef A, & Verseil C (1995) Interlaboratory evaluation of embryotoxicity in the postimplantation rat embryo culture. Reprod Toxicol, **9**: 275–280.

Porcelli F, Redi CA, & Succi G (1984) Chromatin condensation patterns of spermatozoa during epididymal passage in normal and a chimeric bull. Basic Appl Histochem, **28**(2): 159–168.

Pratt RM, Yoneda T, Silver MH, & Salomon DS (1980) Involvement of glucocorticoids and epidermal growth factor in secondary palate development. In: Pratt RM & Christiansen RL ed. Current research trends in prenatal craniofacial development. New York, Elsevier/North-Holland Publishers, pp 235–252.

Pratt RM, Grove RI, & Willis WD (1982) Prescreening for environmental teratogens using cultured mesenchymal cells from the human embryonic palate. Teratog Carcinog Mutagen, **2**: 313–318.

Reinhardt CA (1993) Neurodevelopmental toxicity *in vitro*: Primary cell culture models for screening and risk assessment. Reprod Toxicol, **7**(Suppl 1): 165–170.

Rice JM (1981) Prenatal susceptibility to carcinogenesis by xenobiotic substances including vinyl chloride. Environ Health Perspect, **41**: 179–188.

Rice JM & Wilbourn JD (2000) Tumors of the nervous system in carcinogenic hazard identification. Toxicol Pathol, **28**(1): 202–214.

Rodier PM (1986) Time of exposure and time of testing in developmental neurotoxicology. Neurotoxicology, **7**: 69–76.

Rodier PM (1990) Developmental neurotoxicology. Toxicol Pathol, **18**: 89–95.

Rodriguez H & Bustus-Obregõn E (2000) An *in vitro* model to evaluate the effect of an organophosphoric agropesticide on cell proliferation in mouse seminiferous tubules. Andrologia, **32**: 1–5.

Rogan WJ, Gladen BC, McKinney JD, Carreras N, Hardy P, Thullen J, Tinglestad J, & Tully M (1986) Neonatal effects of transplacental exposure to PCBs and DDE. J Pediatr, **109**: 335–341.

Rogers JM, Taubeneck MW, Daston GP, Sulik KK, Zucker RM, Elstein KH, Jankowski MA, & Keen CL (1995) Zinc deficiency causes apoptosis but not cell cycle alterations in organogenesis-stage rat embryos: effect of varying duration of deficiency. Teratology, **52**(3): 149–159.

Rose RM, Gordon TP, & Bernstein IS (1978) Plasma testosterone levels in male rhesus. Influence of sexual and social stimuli. Science, **178**: 643.

Rothman KJ & Greenland S (1998) Modern epidemiology, 2nd ed. Philadelphia, Pennsylvania, Lippincott-Raven.

Russel LD, Ettlin R, Sinha Hikim AP, & Clegg ED (1990) Histological and histopathological evaluation of the testis. Clearwater, Florida, Cache River Press.

Rutledge JC & Generoso WM (1989) Fetal pathology by ethylene oxide treatment of the murine zygote. Teratology, **39**: 563–572.

Rutledge JC, Generoso WM, Shourbaji A, Cain KT, Gans M, & Oliva J (1992) Developmental anomalies derived from exposure of zygotes and first-cleavage embryos to mutagens. Mutat Res, **296**: 167–177.

Safe SH (2000) Endocrine disruptors and human health — Is there a problem? An update. Environ Health Perspect, **108**: 487–493.

Saleweski E (1964) Farbemethode zum makroskopischen Nachweis von Implantationsstellen am Uterus der Ratte. Naunyn-Schmiedebergs Arch Exp Pathol Pharmakol, **247**: 367.

Samuels SJ (1988) Lessons from a surveillance program of semen quality. Reprod Toxicol, **2**: 229–231.

Sariola H & Sainio K (1998) Cell lineages in the embryonic kidney; their inductive interactions and signallin molecules. Biochem Cell Biol, **76**: 1009–1016.

Sato T, Nonaka K, Miura T, & Peter K (1994) Trends in cohort fertility of the Driusleut Hutterite population. Hum Biol, **66**: 421–431.

Savitz DA (1994) Paternal exposures and pregnancy outcome: miscarriage, stillbirth, low birth weight, preterm delivery. In: Olshan AF & Mattison DR ed. Male-mediated developmental toxicity. New York, Plenum Press, pp 177–196.

Savitz DA & Harlow SD (1991) Selection of reproductive health end points for environmental risk assessment. Environ Health Perspect, 90: 159–164.

Savitz DA, Arbuckle T, Kaczor D, & Curtis KM (1997) Male pesticide exposure and pregnancy outcome. Am J Epidemiol, 146: 1025–1036.

Schardein JL (1993) Chemically induced birth defects, 2nd ed. New York, Marcel Dekker.

Schmid BP, Trippmacher A, & Bianchi A (1982) Teratogenicity induced in cultured rat embryos by the serum of procarbazine treated rats. Toxicology, 25: 53–60.

Schmid BP, Honegger P, & Kucera P (1993) Embryonic and fetal development: Fundamental research. Reprod Toxicol, 7(Suppl 1): 155–164.

Scholz G, Pohl I, Genschow E, Klemm M, & Spielmann H (1999) Embryotoxicity screening using embryonic stem cells in vitro: correlation to in vivo teratogenicity. Cells Tissues Organs, 165: 203–211.

Schwetz BA (1993) In vitro approaches in developmental toxicology. Reprod Toxicol, 7(Suppl 1): 125–127.

Scialli AR, Swan SH, Amier RW, Baird DD, Eskenazi B, Gist G, Hatch MC, Kesner S, Lemasters GK, Marcus M, Paul ME, Schulte P, Taylor Z, Wilcox AJ, & Zahniser C (1997) Assessment of reproductive disorders and birth defects in communities near hazardous chemical sites. II. Female reproductive disorders. Reprod Toxicol, 11: 231–242.

Seed J, Chapin RE, Clegg ED, Dostal LA, Foote RH, Hurtt ME, Klinefelter GR, Makris SI, Perreault SD, Schrader S, Seyler D, Sprando R, Treinen KA, Veeramachaneni DN, & Wise LD (1996) Methods for assessing sperm motility, morphology, and counts in the rat, rabbit and dog: a consensus report. Reprod Toxicol, 10(3): 237–244.

Seibel MM, Shine W, Smith DM, & Taymor ML (1982) Biological rhythm of the luteinizing hormone surge in women. Fertil Steril, 37: 709–711.

Selevan SG (1991) Environmental exposures and reproduction. In: Keily M ed. Reproductive and perinatal epidemiology. Boca Raton, Florida, CRC Press, pp 115–130.

Selevan SG, Kimmel CA, & Mendola P (2000) Identifying critical windows of exposure for children's health. Environ Health Perspect, 108(Suppl 3): 451–455.

Sharpe RM (1993) Falling sperm counts in men — Is there an endocrine cause? J Endocrinol, 137: 357.

Sharpe RM (1994) Regulation of spermatogenesis. In: Knobil E & Neill JD ed. The physiology of reproduction, 2nd ed. New York, Raven Press, pp 1363–1434.

Sharpe RM, Fisher JS, Millar MM, Jobling S, & Sumpter JP (1995) Gestational and lactational exposure of rats to xenoestrogens results in reduced testicular size and sperm production. Environ Health Perspect, 103: 1136–1143.

Shaw G, Wasserman CR, Lammer EJ, O'Malley CD, Murray JC, Basart AM, & Tolarova MM (1996) Orofacial clefts, parental cigarette smoking, and transforming growth factor-alpha gene variants. Am J Hum Genet, 58: 551–561.

Shuey DL, Lau C, Logsdon RR, Zucker RM, Elstein KH, Narotsky MG, Setzer RW, Kavlock RJ, & Rogers JM (1994) Biologically-based dose–response modeling in developmental toxicology: biochemical and cellular sequelae of 5-fluorouracil exposure in the developing rat. Toxicol Appl Pharmacol, **126**: 129–144.

Silbergeld EK (1991) Lead in bone: implications for toxicology during pregnancy and lactation. Environ Health Perspect, **91**: 63–70.

Silbergeld EK, Schwartz J, & Mahaffey K (1988) Lead and osteoporosis: mobilization of lead from bone in postmenopausal women. Environ Res, **47**: 79–94.

Silverman J, Kline J, & Hutzler M (1985) Maternal employment and the chromosomal characteristics of spontaneously aborted conceptions. J Occup Med, **27**: 427–438.

Sipes IG & Gandolfi AJ (1991) Biotransformation of toxicants. In: Amdur MO, Doull J, & Klaassen CD ed. Casarett and Doull's toxicology: The basic science of poisons, 4th ed. New York, McGraw-Hill, pp 13–16.

Slikker W Jr & Miller RK (1994) Placental metabolism and transfer: Role in developmental toxicology. In: Kimmel CA & Buelke-Sam J ed. Developmental toxicology, 2nd ed. New York, Raven Press, pp 245–283.

Sloter E, Lowe X, Moore DH, Nath J, & Wyrobek AJ (2000) Multicolor FISH analysis of chromosomal breaks, duplications, deletions, and numerical abnormalities in the sperm of healthy men. Am J Hum Genet, **67**: 862–872.

Slott VL, Suarez JD, & Perreault SD (1991) Rat sperm motility analysis: Methodologic considerations. Reprod Toxicol, **5**: 449–458.

Slott VL, Jeffay SC, Suarez JD, Barbee RR, & Perreault SD (1995) Synchronous assessment of sperm motility and fertilizing ability in the hamster following treatment with alpha-chlorohydrin. J Androl, **16**: 523–535.

Smart JL & Dobbing J (1971) Vulnerability of developing brain. II. Effects of early nutritional deprivation on reflex ontogeny and development of behaviour in the rat. Brain Res, **28**: 85–95.

Smith BJ, Plowchalk DR, Sipes IG, & Mattison DR (1991) Comparison of random and serial sections in assessment of ovarian toxicity. Reprod Toxicol, **5**: 379–383.

Smith SK, He Y, Clark DE, & Charnock-Jones DS (2000) Angiogenic growth factor expression in placenta. Semin Perinatol, **24**: 82–86.

Snell LM, Little BB, Knoll KA, & Johnston WL (1992) Reliability of birth certificate reporting of congenital anomalies. Am J Perinatol, **9**: 219–222.

Sonawane BR (1995) Chemical contaminants in human milk: an overview. Environ Health Perspect, **103**: 197–205.

Soto AM, Sonnenschein C, Chung KL, Fernandez MF, Olea N, & Serrano FO (1995) The E-Screen assay as a tool to identify estrogens: an update on estrogenic environmental pollutants. Environ Health Perspect, **103**(Suppl 7): 113–122.

Spielmann H, Pohl I, Döring B, Liebsch M, & Moldenhauer F (1997) The embryonic stem cell test (EST), an *in vitro* embryotoxicity test using two permanent mouse cell lines: 3T2 fibroblasts and embryonic stem cells. In Vitro Toxicol, **10**: 119–127.

Spyker JM (1975) Assessing the impact of low level chemicals on development: Behavioral and latent effects. Fed Proc, **34**: 1835–1844.

Stahlmann R, Klug S, Foerster M, & Neubert D (1993) Significance of embryoculture methods for studying the prenatal toxicity of virustatic agents. Reprod Toxicol, **7**(Suppl 1): 129–143.

Stein A & Hatch M (1987) Biological markers in reproductive epidemiology: prospects and precautions. Environ Health, **74**: 67–75.

Stephen EH & Chandra A (1998) Updated projections of infertility in the United States: 1995–2025. Fertil Steril, **70**(1): 30–34.

Stykova A, Chowdhury K, Bonaldo P, Torres M, & Gruss P (1998) Gene trap expression and mutational analysis for genes involved in the development of the mammalian nervous system. Dev Dynam, **212**(2):198–213.

Sullivan FM (1993) Impact of the environment on reproduction from conception to parturition. Environ Health Perspect, **101**(Suppl 2): 13–18.

Susser M (1977) Judgement and causal inference: criteria in epidemiologic studies. Am J Epidemiol, **105**(1): 1–15.

Szabo KT (1989) Congenital malformations in laboratory and farm animals. San Diego, California, Academic Press, p 294.

Tabacova S, Baird DD, & Balabaeva L (1998) Exposure to oxidized nitrogen: Lipid peroxidation and neonatal health risk. Arch Environ Health, **53**: 214–221.

Takano H, Yanagimachi R, & Urch UA (1993) Evidence that acrosin activity is important for the development of fusibility of mammalian spermatozoa with the oolemma: Inhibitor studies using the golden hamster. Zygote, **1**: 79.

Terry KK, Elswick BA, Stedman DB, & Welsch F (1994) Developmental phase alters dosimetry–teratogenicity relationship for 2-methoxyethanol in CD-1 mice. Teratology, **49**: 218–227.

Testart J, Frydman R, & Roger M (1982) Seasonal influence of dirunal rhythms in onset of plasma luteinizing hormone surge in women. J Clin Exp Metabol, **55**: 374–377.

Thomas JA (1981) Reproductive hazards and environmental chemicals: a review. Toxic Subst J, **2**: 318–348.

Thonneau P, Abell A, Larsen SB, Bonde JP, Joffe M, Clavert A, Ducot B, Multinger L, & Danscher G (1999) Effects of pesticide exposure on time to pregnancy: results of a multicenter study in France and Denmark. ASCLEPIOS Study Group. Am J Epidemiol, **150**: 157–163.

Tilson HA (1990) Behavioural indices of neurotoxicity. Toxicol Pathol, **18**: 96–104.

Tilson HA (1998) The concern for developmental neurotoxicology: Is it justified and what is being done about it? Environ Health Perspect, **103**: 147–151.

Tilson H & Mitchell C (1980) Models for neurotoxicity. In: Hodgson E, Bend J, & Philpot R ed. Reviews in biomedical toxicology. New York, Elsevier/North-Holland, pp 265–294.

Tilson HA, MacPhail RC, Moser VC, Becking GC, Cuomo V, Frantik E, Kulig BM, & Winneke G (1997) The IPCS collaborative study on neurobehavioural screening methods: VII. Summary and conclusions. Neurotoxicology, **18**(4): 1065–1069.

Toppari J, Lahdetie J, Harkonen P, Eerola E, & Parvinen M (1986) Mutagen effects on rat seminiferous tubules *in vitro*: induction of meiotic micronuclei by adriamycin. Mutat Res, **171**(2–3): 149–156.

Toppari J, Bishop PC, Parker JW, Ahmad N, Girgis W, & diZerega GS (1990) Cytotoxic effects of cyclophosphamide in the mouse seminiferous epithelium: DNA flow cytometric and morphometric analysis. Fundam Appl Toxicol, **15**: 44–52.

Toppari J, Larsen JC, Christiansen P, Giwercman A, Grandjean P, Guillette LJ Jr, Jegou B, Jensen TK, Jouannet P, Keiding N, Leffers H, McLachlan JA, Meyer O, Muller J, Rajpert-De Meyts E, Scheike T, Sharpe R, Sumpter J, & Skakkebaek NE (1996) Male reproductive health and environmental xenoestrogens. Environ Health Perspect, **104**(Suppl 4): 741–776.

Torres M, Gomez-Pardo E, Dressler GR, & Gruss P (1995) Pax-2 controls multiple steps of urogenital development. Development, **121**(12): 4057–4065.

Toth GP, Stober JA, George EL, Read EJ, & Smith MK (1991a) Sources of variation in the computer-assisted motion analysis of rat epididymal sperm. Reprod Toxicol, **5**: 487–495.

Toth GP, Stober JA, Zenich H, Read EJ, Christ SA, & Smith MK (1991b) Correlation of sperm motion parameters with fertility in rats treated subchronically with epichlorohydrin. J Androl, **12**: 54–61.

Treloar AE, Boynton RW, Borghild GB, & Brown BW (1967) Variation in the human menstrual cycle through reproductive life. Int J Fertil, **12**: 77–126.

Tres LL, Smith EP, Van Wyk KK, & Kierszenbaum AL (1986) Immunoreactive sites and accumulation of somatomedin-C in rat Sertoli–spermatogenic cell co-cultures. Exp Cell Res, **162**(1): 33–50.

Tsafriri A & Adashi EY (1994) Local nonsteroidal regulators of ovarian function. In: Knobil E & Neill JD ed. The physiology of reproduction, 2nd ed. Vol. 1. New York, Raven Press, p 817.

Tsonis CG, Hiller SG, & Baird DT (1987) Production of inhibin bioactivity by human granulosa-lutein cells: Stimulation by LH and testosterone *in vitro*. J Endocrinol, **112**: R11–R14.

Tucker HA (1994) Lactation and its hormonal control. In: Adashi EY, Rock JA, & Rosenwaks Z ed. Reproductive endocrinology, surgery, and technology. Philadelphia, Pennsylvania, Lippincott-Raven Publishers, pp 1065–1098.

United Kingdom Department of Health (1991) Committee on Carcinogenicity of Chemicals in Food, Consumer Products and the Environment: Guidelines for the evaluation of chemicals for carcinogenicity. London, Her Majesty's Stationery Office.

United Kingdom Department of Health (1995) Annual report of the Committees on Toxicity, Mutagenicity, Carcinogenicity of Chemicals in Food, Consumer Products and the Environment. London, Her Majesty's Stationery Office.

US EPA (1986) Pesticide products containing dinoseb; notices. US Environmental Protection Agency. Fed Regist, **51**: 36645–36661.

US EPA (1991) Guidelines for the developmental toxicity risk assessment; notice. US Environmental Protection Agency. Fed Regist, **56**: 63798–63826.

US EPA (1992) Guidelines for exposure assessment; notice. US Environmental Protection Agency. Fed Regist, **57**: 22888–22938.

US EPA (1995) The use of the benchmark dose approach in health risk assessment. Washington, DC, US Environmental Protection Agency (EPA/630/R-94-007).

US EPA (1996a) The Safe Drinking Water Act Amendments and Food Quality Protection Act, 1996. Washington, DC, US Environmental Protection Agency.

US EPA (1996b) Guidelines for reproductive toxicity risk assessment. US Environmental Protection Agency. Fed Regist, **61**: 56274–56322.

US EPA (1996c) Draft benchmark dose technical guidance document. Washington, DC, US Environmental Protection Agency (EPA/600/P-96/002A).

US EPA (1997a) Exposure factors handbook — final report. Washington, DC, US Environmental Protection Agency (EPA/600P-95/002Bc).

US EPA (1997b) Special report on environmental endocrine disruption: An effects assessment and analysis. Washington, DC, US Environmental Protection Agency, Office of Research and Development (EPA/630/R-96/012).

US EPA (1998a) Health effects test guidelines OPPTS 870.3800: Reproduction and fertility. Washington, DC, US Environmental Protection Agency (EPA 712-C-98-208).

US EPA (1998b) Health effects test guidelines OPPTS 870.3700: Prenatal developmental toxicity. Washington, DC, US Environmental Protection Agency (EPA 712-C-98-207).

US EPA (1998c) Health effects test guidelines OPPTS 870.6300: Developmental neurotoxicity. Washington, DC, US Environmental Protection Agency (EPA 712-C-98-239).

US EPA (1998d) Endocrine Disruptor Screening and Testing Advisory Committee (EDSTAC) final report. Washington, DC, US Environmental Protection Agency.

US FDA (1966) Guidelines for reproduction studies for safety evaluation of drugs for human use. Rockville, Maryland, US Food and Drug Administration.

US FDA (1970) Guidelines for food additives and contaminants. Rockville, Maryland, US Food and Drug Administration.

US FDA (1982) Toxicological principles for the safety assessment of direct food additives and color additives used in food ("Redbook"). Rockville, Maryland, US Food and Drug Administration.

US FDA (1993) Draft revised toxicological principles for the safety assessment of direct food additives and color additives used in food ("Redbook II"). Rockville, Maryland, US Food and Drug Administration.

US NRC (1983) Risk assessment in the federal government: Managing the process. Committee on the Institutional Means for the Assessment of Risks to Public Health, Commission on Life Sciences. Washington, DC, US National Research Council, National Academy Press.

US NRC (1991) Environmental epidemiology. Committee on Environmental Epidemiology. Washington, DC, US National Research Council, National Academy Press.

US NRC (1993) Pesticides in the diets of infants and children. Washington, DC, US National Research Council, National Academy Press.

US NRC (1999) Hormonally active agents in the environment. Washington, DC, US National Research Council, National Academy Press.

US NRC (2000) Scientific frontiers in developmental toxicology and risk assessment. Washington, DC, US National Research Council, National Academy Press.

Vale VW, Bilezikjian LM, & Rivier C (1994) Inhibins and activins. In: Knobil E & Neill JD ed. The physiology of reproduction, 2nd ed. New York, Raven Press, pp 1861–1878.

Vandenbergh JG & Vessey S (1968) Seasonal breeding of free ranging rhesus monkeys and related ecological factors. J Reprod Fertil, **15**: 71–79.

van der Pal-de Bruin KM, Verloove-Vanhorick SP, & Roeleveld N (1997) Change in male:female ratio among newborn babies in Netherlands. Lancet, **349**: 62.

Van Maele-Fabry G, Picard JJ, Attenon P, Berthet B, Delhaise F, Govers MJAP, Peters PWJ, Piersma AH, Schmid BP, Stadler J, Verhoef A, & Verseil C (1991) Interlaboratory evaluation of three culture media for postimplantation rodent embryos. Reprod Toxicol, **5**: 417–426.

Van Vugt DA (1990) Influences of the visual and olfactory systems on reproduction. Semin Reprod Endocrinol, **8**: 1–7.

Vartianen T, Kartovaara L, & Tuomisto J (1999) Environmental chemicals and changes in sex ratio: analysis over 250 years in Finland. Environ Health Perspect, **107**: 813–815.

Vermeulen A (1993) Environmental, human reproduction, menopause, and andropause. Environ Health Perspect, **101**(Suppl 2): 91–100.

Vorhees CV (1986) Principles of behavioural teratology. In: Riley EP & Voorhees CV ed. Handbook of behavioural teratology. New York, Plenum Press, pp 23–66.

Walker CH (1978) Species differences in microsomal monooxygenase activity and their relationship to biological half-lives. Drug Metab Rev, **7**: 295–323.

Walker CH (1986) Age factors potentiating drug toxicity in the reproductive axis. Environ Health, **70**: 185–191.

Waller CL & McKinney JD (1995) Three-dimensional quantitative structure activity relationships of dioxins and dioxin-like compounds: Model validation and Ah receptor characterization. Chem Res Toxicol, **8**: 847–858.

Waller CL, Juma BW, Gray JE Jr, & Kelce WE (1996) Three-dimensional quantitative structure activity relationships for androgen receptor ligands. Toxicol Appl Pharmacol, **137**: 219–227.

Warren JC, Cheatum SG, Greenwald GS, & Barker KL (1967) Cyclic variation of uterine metabolic activity in the golden hamster. Endocrinology, **80**: 714–718.

Wasserman PM (1996) Oogenesis. In: Adashi EY, Rock JA, & Rosenwaks Z ed. Reproductive endocrinology, surgery, and technology. Philadelphia, Pennsylvania, Lippincott-Raven, pp 342–357.

Wasserman PM & Albertini DF (1996) The mammalian ovum. In: Adashi EY, Rock JA, & Rosenwaks Z ed. Reproductive endocrinology, surgery, and technology. Philadelphia, Pennsylvania, Lippincott-Raven, pp 79–122.

Watson LR, Gandley R, & Silbergeld EK (1993) Lead: interactions of pregnancy and lactation with lead exposure in rats. Toxicologist, **13**: 349–356.

Webster WS, Johnston MC, Lammer EJ, & Sulik KK (1986) Isotretinoin embryopathy and the cranial neural crest: an *in vivo* and *in vitro* study. J Craniofac Genet Dev Biol, 6(3): 211–222.

Weidner IS, Moller H, Jensen TK, & Skakkebaek NE (1999) Risk factors for cryptorchidism and hypospadias. J Urol, **161**: 1606–1609.

Weinberg CR & Gladen BC (1986) The beta-geometric distribution applied to comparative fecundability studies. Biometrics, **42**: 547–560.

Weinberg CR & Wilcox AJ (1998) Reproductive epidemiology. In: Rothman KJ & Greenland S ed. Modern epidemiology, 2nd ed. Philadelphia, Pennsylvania, Lippincott-Raven, pp 585–608.

Weinberg CR, Baird DD, & Wilcox AJ (1994) Sources of bias in studies of time to pregnancy. Stat Med, **13**: 671–681.

Weiss B (1975) Effects on behavior. In: Principles for evaluating chemicals in the environment. Washington, DC, US National Research Council, National Academy of Sciences, pp 198–216.

Weiss B (2000) Vulnerability of children and the developing brain to neurotoxic hazards. Environ Health Perspect, **108**(Suppl 3): 375–381.

Welch LS, Plotkin E, & Schrader S (1991) Indirect fertility analysis in painters exposed to ethylene glycol ethers: Sensitivity and specificity. Am J Ind Med, **20**: 229–240.

Welsch F (1990) Short term methods of assessing developmental toxicity hazard. In: Kalter H ed. Issues and reviews in teratology, Vol. 5. New York, Plenum Press, pp 115–153.

Werboff J & Gottlieb JS (1963) Drugs in pregnancy: Behavioural teratology. Obstet Gynecol Surv, **18**: 420–427.

Whitaker J & Dix KM (1979) Double staining techniques for rat foetus skeletons in teratological studies. Lab Anim, **13**: 309–310.

WHO (1967) Principles for the testing of drugs for teratogenicity. Geneva, World Health Organization (Technical Report Series 364).

WHO (1988) Assessment of health risks in infants associated with exposure to PCBs, PCDDs and PCDFs in breast milk. Copenhagen, World Health Organization (Environmental Health Series No. 29).

WHO (1995) Guidelines for good clinical practice for trials on pharmaceutical products. Geneva, World Health Organization (WHO Technical Report Series No. 850).

WHO (1999) WHO laboratory manual for the examination of human semen and sperm–cervical mucus interaction, 4th ed. Cambridge, Cambridge University Press, and Geneva, World Health Organization.

Whorton D, Krauss RM, Marshall S, & Milby TH (1977) Infertility in male pesticide workers [preliminary communication]. Lancet, 2(8051): 1259–1261.

Whorton D, Milby TH, Krauss RM, & Stubbs HA (1979) Testicular function in DBCP exposed pesticide workers. J Occup Med, 21: 161–166.

Wilcox AJ (1983) Surveillance of pregnancy loss in human populations. Am J Ind Med, 4: 285–291.

Wilcox AJ, Weinberg CR, Wehmann RE, Armstrong EG, Canfield RE, & Nisula BC (1985) Measuring early pregnancy loss: laboratory and field methods. Fertil Steril, 44: 366–374.

Wilcox AJ, Baird DD, & Weinberg CR (1999) Time of implantation of the conceptus and loss of pregnancy. N Engl J Med, 340(23): 1796–1799.

Wilkie AO, Amberger JS, & McKusick VA (1994) A gene map of congenital malformations. J Med Genet, 31(7): 507–517.

Williams J, Gladen BC, Schrader SM, Turner TW, Phelps JL, & Chapin RE (1990) Semen analysis and fertility assessment in rabbits: Statistical power and design considerations for toxicology studies. Fundam Appl Toxicol, 15: 651–665.

Wilson JG (1965) Methods for administering agents and detecting malformations in experimental animals. In: Wilson JG & Warkany J ed. Teratology: Principles and techniques. Chicago, Illinois, University of Chicago Press, pp 262–277.

Wine RN, Li LH, Gulati DK, & Chapin RE (1997) Reproductive toxicity of di-*n*-butylphthalate in a continuous breeding protocol in Sprague-Dawley rats. Environ Health Perspect, 105(1): 102–107.

Winneke G (1995) Endpoints of developmental neurotoxicity in environmentally exposed children. Toxicol Lett, 77(1–3): 127–136.

Wise LD, Beck SL, Beltrame D, Beyer BK, Chahoud I, Clark RL, Clark R, Druga AM, Feuston MH, Guittin P, Henwood SM, Kimmel CA, Lindstrom P, Palmer AK, Petrere JA, Solomon HM, Yasuda M, & York RG (1997) Terminology of developmental abnormalities in common laboratory mammals (version 1). Teratology, 55: 249–292.

Wolff MS (1993) Lactation. In: Paul M ed. Occupational and environmental reproductive hazards. Baltimore, Maryland, Williams & Wilkins, pp 60–75.

Wolpert L & Brown NA (1995) Developmental biology; hedgehog keeps to the left. Nature, 6545: 103–104.

Working PK (1988) Male reproductive toxicity: comparison of the human to animal models. Environ Health, 77: 37–44.

Working PK & Hurtt ME (1987) Computerized videomicrographic analysis of rat sperm motility. J Androl, **8**: 330–337.

Wyrobek AJ (1982) Sperm assays as indicators of chemically-induced germ cell damage in man. In: Heddle JA ed. Mutagenicity: New horizons in genetic toxicology. New York, Academic Press, pp 337–349.

Wyrobek AJ (1984) Identifying agents that damage human spermatogenesis: abnormalities in sperm concentration and morphology. In: Monitoring human exposure to carcinogenic and mutagenic agents. Proceedings of a joint symposium held in Espoo, Finland, 12–15 December 1983. Lyon, International Agency for Research on Cancer.

Wyrobek AJ, Gordon LA, Burkhart JG, Francis MW, Kapp RW, Letz G, Malling HV, Topham JC, & Whorton DM (1983) An evaluation of human sperm as indicators of chemically induced alterations of spermatogenic function. Mutat Res, **115**: 73–148.

Yanagimachi R (1970) The movement of golden hamster spermatozoa before and after capacitation. J Reprod Fertil, **23**: 193–196.

Yanagimachi R (1988) Sperm–egg fusion. Curr Topics Membrane Transport, **32**: 349–363.

Yanagimachi R, Yanagimachi H, & Rogers BJ (1976) The use of zona-free animal ova as a test-system for the assessment of the fertilizing capacity of human spermatozoa. Biol Reprod, **15**: 471–476.

Zenick H, Blackburn K, Hope E, & Baldwin DJ (1984) Evaluating male reproductive toxicity in rodents: A new animal model. Teratog Carcinog Mutagen, **4**: 109–128.

Zinaman MJ, Clegg ED, Brown CC, O'Connor J, & Selevan SG (1996) Estimates of human fertility and pregnancy loss. Fertil Steril, **65**(3): 503–509.

APPENDIX: TERMINOLOGY

This appendix provides working definitions for selected terms as used in this document. These definitions are not necessarily valid for other purposes.

Acceptable daily intake: The maximum amount of a substance to which a subject may be exposed daily over a lifetime without appreciable health risk.

Adolescence: The period of life beginning with the appearance of secondary sex characteristics and terminating with full maturity.

Adverse effect: A treatment-related alteration from baseline that diminishes an organism's ability to survive, reproduce or adapt to the environment.

Altered sexual function and fertility: Toxicity may be expressed as alterations to the female or male reproductive organs, the related endocrine system or pregnancy outcomes. The manifestations of such toxicity may include, but not be limited to, adverse effects on onset of puberty, gamete production and transport, reproductive cycle normality, sexual behaviour, fertility, gestation, parturition, lactation, pregnancy outcomes, premature reproductive senescence or modifications in other functions that are dependent on the integrity of the reproductive systems.

Anomalies: Marked deviation from the normal standard.

Azoospermia: Less than the reference value for morphology of spermatozoa.

Congenital malformation: A permanent structural abnormality.

Critical period: A specific phase during which a developing system is particularly vulnerable.

Developmental disorders: Adverse effects on the developing organism that may result from exposure prior to conception (either parent), during prenatal development or postnatally to the time of sexual maturation. Adverse developmental effects may be detected at any point in the life span of the organism.

Developmental toxicity: Taken in its widest sense to include any effect interfering with normal development both before and after birth. The occurrence of adverse effects in the developing organism may result from exposure of either parent prior to conception, exposure during prenatal development or exposure postnatally to the time of sexual maturation. Adverse developmental effects may be detected at any point in the life span of the organism.

Dose (exposure)–response relationship: Characterization of the relationship between administered dose or exposure and the biological change in organisms. It may be expressed as the severity of an effect in one organism (or part of an organism) or as the proportion of a population exposed to a chemical that shows a specific reaction.

Embryo: The early or developing stage of any organism, especially the developing product of fertilization of an egg.

Embryonic period: The period from fertilization to the end of major organogenesis.

Embryotoxicity (Fetotoxicity): Injury to the embryo (fetus), which may result in death or abnormal development or growth alteration.

Endocrine disrupting chemicals: Exogenous chemicals that alter function(s) of the endocrine system and consequently cause adverse health effects in an intact organism, its progeny or (sub)populations.

Exposure assessment: The qualitative and/or quantitative assessment of the chemical nature, form and concentration of a chemical to which an identified population is exposed from all sources (air, water, soil and diet).

Fecundity: The ability to produce offspring within a given period of time. For litter-bearing species, the ability to produce large litters is also a component of fecundity.

Fertility: The capacity to become pregnant or to impregnate. In humans, the capacity for producing viable offspring.

Fertilization: The fusion of the sperm and ovum resulting in the restoration of the diploid number of chromosomes.

Fetal period: The period from the end of embryogenesis to the completion of pregnancy.

Gestation: Length of time between conception and birth.

Hazard characterization: Involves determining whether or not an agent poses a hazard, at what doses and under what conditions of exposure.

Hazard identification: The identification of the inherent capability of a substance to cause adverse effects.

Implantation: Attachment of the fertilized ovum (blastocyst) to the endometrium and its subsequent embedding in the compact layer, occurring 6 or 7 days after fertilization of the ovum.

Infant: A child under the age of 1 year.

Infertility: Inability to become pregnant within 1 year of unprotected intercourse.

Lowest-observed-adverse-effect level (LOAEL): The lowest concentration or amount of a substance, found by experiment or observation, that causes an adverse alteration of morphology, functional capacity, growth, development or life span of the target organism distinguishable from normal (control) organisms of the same species and strain under the same defined conditions of exposure.

Lowest-observed-effect level (LOEL): The lowest concentration or amount of a substance, found by experiment or observation, that causes any alteration in morphology, functional capacity, growth, development or life span of the target organism distinguishable from normal (control) organisms of the same species and strain under the same defined conditions of exposure.

Margin of exposure: The ratio of the NOAEL to the estimated exposure dose.

Neonate: Newborn baby, from immediately after birth through the first 28 days of life.

No-observed-adverse-effect level (NOAEL): Highest concentration or amount of a substance, found by experiment or observation, that causes no detectable adverse alteration of morphology, functional capacity, growth, development or life span of the target organism under defined conditions of exposure. Alterations of morphology, functional capacity, growth, development or life span of the target organism may be detected that are not judged to be adverse.

No-observed-effect level (NOEL): Highest concentration or amount of a substance, found by experiment or observation, that causes no alterations of morphology, functional capacity, growth, development or life span of the target organism distinguishable from those observed in normal (control) organisms of the same species and strain under the same defined conditions of exposure.

Oligozoospermia: Sperm concentration less than the reference value.

Perinatal: The period before, during and after the time of birth, i.e., before delivery from the 28th week of gestation through the first 7 days after delivery.

Pregnancy: The condition of having an implanted embryo or fetus in the body, after fusion of an ovum and spermatozoon.

Premature ovarian failure: Follicular depletion by the age of 35 years.

Risk assessment: An empirically based paradigm that estimates the risk of adverse effect(s) from exposure of an individual or population to a chemical, physical or biological agent. It includes the components of hazard identification, assessment of dose–response relationships, exposure assessment and risk characterization.

Risk characterization: The synthesis of critically evaluated information and data from exposure assessment, hazard identification and dose–response considerations into a summary that identifies clearly the strengths and weaknesses of the database, the criteria applied to evaluation and validation of all aspects of methodology and the conclusions reached from the review of scientific information.

Sexual maturation: Achievement of full development of sexual function and reproductive system.

Subfertility: Fertility below the normal range for that species.

Teratogenicity: Induction of structural abnormality.

RESUME ET RECOMMANDATIONS

1. Résumé

Depuis la publication au début des années 1980 des documents IPCS de la série *Critères d'hygiène de l'environnement* relatifs à l'évaluation des risques de toxicité pour la fonction de reproduction, de nouvelles données et méthodes scientifiques ont fait leur apparition, qui permettent de déterminer sensiblement mieux de quelle manière des substances chimiques sont susceptibles d'exercer des effets nocifs sur l'appareil reproducteur. Ces progrès transparaissent dans l'existence d'un certain nombre de principes directeurs d'origine nationale ou internationale (par ex. ceux de l'Organisation de coopération et de développement économiques - OCDE) applicables à l'évaluation des effets toxiques sur la reproduction et le développement ou à l'évaluation des risques en général, de documents d'orientation ou encore de quelques études internationales pour la validation des méthodes d'épreuve. Quoi qu'il en soit, le risque d'exposition humaine aux polluants présents dans l'environnement (par diverses voies), avec ses conséquences pour l'appareil reproducteur et le développement, demeure un sujet de préoccupation au niveau mondial.

Dans les conditions normales, la reproduction humaine est régulée par un système extrêmement pointu de signaux coordonnés qui commandent l'activité de multiples cellules cibles interdépendantes ayant pour finalité de former des gamètes, d'assurer leur transport, leur libération, leur fécondation, leur implantation et enfin la gestation elle-même, qui aboutira au développement d'une progéniture également capable, le moment venu, de reprendre la totalité du processus dans des conditions environnementales analogues ou différentes.

Tout au long de l'existence, la fonction de reproduction dans son ensemble est tributaire de divers systèmes de communication endocrines utilisant toute une variété de protéines, de peptides, d'hormones stéroïdiennes, de facteurs de croissance ou d'autres molécules de signalisation qui agissent sur l'expression des gènes ou la synthèse des protéines au niveau des cellules cibles. En particulier, le développement et la gamétogénèse sont régulés par une myriade de signaux qui sont émis avec l'intensité appropriée à des moments parfaitement définis. Des études récentes sur l'animal montrent que l'organisme du foetus en développement pourrait être plus sensible que celui de l'adulte aux substances chimiques présentes dans l'environnement, mais les effets peuvent ne pas se manifester avant l'âge adulte. Il est capital de parvenir à une description plus précise de la régulation normale des divers aspects de la reproduction au niveau moléculaire pour comprendre la variété des mécanismes par lesquels des substances exogènes peuvent désorganiser le cours normal de la reproduction et du développement.

L'activité sexuelle et la fécondité résultent d'un grand nombre de fonctions indispensables à la reproduction qui peuvent être perturbées en cas d'exposition à certains facteurs environnementaux. Toute atteinte à l'intégrité de l'appareil reproducteur peut affecter ces fonctions. Selon les statistiques, la stérilité présente une fréquence variable dans le monde mais environ 10 % des couples passent par une phase de stérilité au cours de leur vie procréative. C'est par l'étude des anomalies de la fonction sexuelle et de la fertilité chez l'Homme que l'on peut évaluer le risque le plus directement, mais les données font souvent défaut. Pour beaucoup de substances chimiques présentes dans l'environnement, il est encore nécessaire de s'appuyer sur les données obtenues sur des modèles animaux ou tirées d'études en laboratoire.

Pour évaluer *in vivo* le risque d'effets toxiques sur la reproduction, on a habituellement recours à des rongeurs de laboratoire. La baisse de la fécondité des animaux mâles n'est pas un indicateur très sensible d'une atteinte de l'appareil reproducteur car chez la plupart des espèces utilisées en laboratoire, les mâles produisent beaucoup plus de spermatozoïdes que le minimum nécessaire pour assurer une fécondité normale. L'évaluation du risque de toxicité génésique chez les mâles repose en grande partie sur l'examen histopathologique des tissus de l'appareil reproducteur. On a mis en évidence, dans le cas de certaines substances chimiques, une activité estrogénique ou anti-androgénique qui les rend capables d'avoir une effet sur la fonction de reproduction chez le mâle. Il peut y avoir des différences de sensibilité, mais il est probable que chez les mammifères, le mode d'action de ces agents perturbateurs du système endocrine est constant ou du moins similaire d'une espèce à l'autre. Dans le cas de la femelle, toutes les fonctions de l'appareil reproducteur sont sous contrôle endocrine et peuvent être perturbées par les effets exercés sur ce système. Toutefois, étant donné la grande variabilité qui existe à l'état normal chez les femelles, un dosage hormonal à la recherche de modifications à ce niveau peut ne pas constituer un indicateur sensible d'une lésion.

Il existe divers systèmes d'épreuve *in vitro* - notamment des testicules ou des ovaires isolés que l'on perfuse, des cultures primaires de cellules gonadiques, l'examen des fractions infracellulaires provenant de différents organes ou de différentes cellules ou encore les techniques de fécondation *in vitro* - qui peuvent être utilisés à titre complémentaire pour l'étude des différents éléments de l'appareil reproducteur. Ces systèmes d'épreuve *in vitro* sont particulièrement utiles pour la rechercher la toxicité éventuelle d'une substance et mettre en évidence les mécanismes par lesquels cette toxicité pourrait s'exercer. Il reste que ces épreuves ont leur limites, notamment lorsqu'il s'agit d'évaluer les fonctions intégrées complexes de l'appareil reproducteur.

Les effets toxiques sur le développement - on parle aussi de *toxicité développementale* - dans leur acception la plus large, c'est-à-dire comprenant tous les effets nocifs qui s'exercent sur le développement avant ou après la naissance, ne cessent de capter l'attention depuis quelques années. Ce type de toxicité peut résulter d'une exposition de l'un ou l'autre des parents avant la conception, d'une exposition *in utero* de l'embryon ou du foetus ou encore une exposition après la naissance. Ces effets peuvent être decelés à n'importe quel moment de l'existence d'un organisme. Outre des anomalies de structure, cette toxicité peut également se manifester par la mort du foetus, un retard de croissance, des troubles fonctionnels, l'apparition tardive d'une maladie à l'âge adulte, la sénescence précoce de l'appareil reproducteur ou une durée de vie plus courte.

On fait largement appel à des études *in vivo* sur des animaux de laboratoire ou leur progéniture pour évaluer les effets toxiques des substances chimiques sur le développement. Par des observations sur la mère, on s'efforce de déterminer quel est la part relative de la toxicité maternelle dans celle que l'on peut observer chez l'embryon ou le foetus. En ce qui concerne la progéniture, les observations consistent à noter la mort à un stade précoce ou tardif de l'embryon (résorptions), le poids du foetus et son sexe, la présence de malformations externes et d'anomalies viscerales ou squelettiques. Pour une interprétation correcte des résultats de ces études toxicologiques, il est important de disposer de données de base et d'archives concernant les anomalies de développement constatées chez les animaux de laboratoire utilisés. Les paramètres susceptibles d'être étudiés après la naissance sont notamment le développement neurologique, les comportements élémentaires ou complexes, la reproduction, les fonctions endocrines, l'immunocompétence, le métabolisme de substances xénobiotiques, et les fonctions physiologiques des divers organes et appareils. Parmi les manifestations latentes de ce type de toxicité on peut également citer la cancérogénicité transplacentaire (apparition de néoplasmes dans la progéniture par suite d'une exposition maternelle à des substances chimiques pendant la gestation) ou la réduction de la durée de vie. On a également mis au point, pour l'étude des effets toxiques sur le développement, des systèmes d'épreuve *in vitro* très variés qui vont de la culture d'embryons entiers à toutes sortes de systèmes non mammaliens, en passant par les cultures d'organes et de tissus. L'utilité des épreuves *in vitro* dans l'étude des mécanismes du développement et de ses anomalies, réside dans le fait qu'elles permettent d'obtenir des informations sur les relations dose-réponse et la toxicité vis-à-vis de tel ou tel organe particulier et le cas échéant, dans la possibilité de s'en servir pour le tri des produits chimiques à évaluer ou l'établissement de listes de priorité en vue d'autres études *in vivo*.

Lorsque l'on se propose d'évaluer les effets toxiques d'une substance sur le développement humain, le point d'aboutissement le plus commode à observer est l'état des fonctions vitales à la naissance (y compris la mort embryonnaire ou foetale), les anomalies congénitales immédiatement reconnaissables, la durée de la gestation, le poids de naissance et le rapport de masculinité. Après la naissance, on peut évaluer les effets sur le développement en étudiant les modifications de la courbe de croissance, du comportement ou des fonctions organiques ou en recherchant la présence éventuelle d'un cancer. Il est possible que les effets anténatals ou postnatals n'apparaissent que bien après la naissance et parfois même pas avant l'âge adulte. Ainsi, certaines anomalies congénitales ne sont pas immédiatement visibles et l'on commence tout juste à se rendre compte des séquelles à long terme d'un retard de croissance intrautérin. Une exposition à des substances chimiques pendant le développement peut également avoir des répercussions sur la fonction de reproduction de la progéniture. Par exemple, ces substances peuvent endommager les cellules germinales femelles *in utero* et par conséquent affecter la fécondité de la femelle ou de la femme parvenue à maturité; de même, il peut y avoir déplétion des cellules souches ou des cellules de Sertoli chez le mâle ou le sujet de sexe masculin, ce qui est susceptible d'entraver la production de spermatozoïdes.

De nombreux pays ont mis au point des procédures d'évaluation du risque de toxicité génésique et développementale afin de fixer des normes et de réglementer l'exposition. Ces procédures comportent le plus souvent les phases suivantes : identification des dangers, établissement de la relation dose-réponse, évaluation de l'exposition et caractérisation du risque. Les protocoles expérimentaux reposent en grande partie sur la mise en évidence d'anomalies de structure et d'insuffisances fonctionnelles consécutives à une exposition à des substances chimiques à certaines périodes critiques du cycle reproductif. L'évaluation d'effets toxiques déterminés sur la reproduction ou le développement doit comporter la consultation de toutes les sources existantes de données toxicologiques sur l'Homme et l'animal. Les méthodes d'évaluation et de synthèse des données de toxicité génésique ont fait des progrès. Il est cependant fréquent que l'évaluation d'un risque comporte une part d'hypothèses en raison des lacunes qui peuvent subsister dans la connaissance des processus biologiques sous-jacents et des différences entre espèces. Les méthodes et les stratégies expérimentales d'évaluation du risque doivent donc être continuellement affinées à mesure qu'apparaissent des données et des technologies nouvelles.

. Recommandations

Pour pouvoir mettre en oeuvre des stratégies efficaces de contrôle et d'intervention destinées à prévenir les effets toxiques sur la reproduction et le développement, il est nécessaire de mettre sur pied une base de connaissances appropriée. Afin d'améliorer cette base de connaissances, il est recommandé :

1. De rechercher et de mettre au point de meilleurs marqueurs (moléculaires) des effets toxiques sur la reproduction et le développement. Ceux qui pourraient être concordants chez l'Homme et l'animal seraient particulièrement utiles et faciliteraient l'évaluation des données animales en vue de leur utilisation pour évaluer le risque chez l'Homme.

2. De voir quelle peut être l'utilité des technologies récentes relatives à l'expression des gènes (« arrays » de gènes, protéomique, microscopie à capture laser, etc.) pour faciliter la compréhension et l'élucidation des mécanismes fondamentaux de la fonction de reproduction et du développemement dans des conditions normales ou anormales.

3. De perfectionner et d'affiner les méthodes permettant de déterminer quelles sont les phases critiques d'exposition pendant tout le cours du développement et quels stades de ce développement sont les plus vulnérables aux manifestations des effets indésirables.

4. De développer les connaissances fondamentales sur les mécanismes physiologiques de la fonction de reproduction chez l'homme et l'animal mâle pour qu'elles atteignent un niveau comparable à celui des connaissances en physiologie de la reproduction chez la femme et les femelles d'animaux.

5. De s'appuyer davantage sur les bases moléculaires et cellulaires de la fonction des gonades et des gamètes pour mieux comprendre la nature des effets toxiques sur ces tissus.

6. De rechercher des modèles animaux et de procéder à leur validation en vue d'analyser les aspects toxicologiques de la biologie de la reproduction et de mettre au point des systèmes expérimentaux qui soient reproductibles, peu coûteux et permettent une extrapolation facile aux pathologies humaines.

7. D'améliorer et de valider les méthodes *in vitro* en vue de déterminer le mode d'action des substances chimiques potentiellement toxiques pour la fonction de reproduction.

8. De mettre au point des méthodes plus précises et plus efficaces pour l'évaluation de l'exposition humaine aux substances chimiques présentes dans l'environnement qui sont potentiellement toxiques pour la fonction de reproduction.

9. D'améliorer la surveillance, la collecte et l'harmonisation des données relatives à la fréquence et à la distribution géographique des anomalies congénitales et des troubles du développement, en

veillant tout particulièrement à l'établissement de registres complets.

10. D'encourager l'effort de recherche afin de mieux identifier les sous-populations qui pourraient être vulnérables aux effets des agents toxiques pour la fonction de reproduction et de caractériser les facteurs qui contribuent à accroître cette vulnérabilité.

11. En raison de la sensibilité de l'organisme en développement, de privilégier les études toxicologiques portant sur l'exposition à tel ou tel produit ou mélange de produits chimiques pendant la période de gestation et la période périnatale.

12. D'utiliser des cohortes de naissance ayant déjà fait l'objet d'études antérieures pour évaluer à un stade ultérieur de l'existence, l'incidence des effets nocifs latents sur la reproduction (les cohortes pour lesquelles on dispose de données d'exposition pendant la grossesse sont extrêmement importantes).

13. D'établir un système international pour l'harmonisation de la terminologie et des définitions relatives aux effets toxiques sur la reproduction et le développement.

RESUMEN Y RECOMENDACIONES

1. Resumen

Desde la publicación de los documentos de los Criterios de Salud Ambiental del IPCS relativos a los aspectos de la evaluación del riesgo de toxicidad reproductiva a comienzos de los años ochenta, los nuevos datos científicos y las nuevas metodologías han introducido mejoras considerables en la capacidad para evaluar la manera en que las sustancias químicas presentes en el medio ambiente pueden afectar negativamente al sistema reproductivo. Este avance se pone de manifiesto en la posibilidad de disponer de varias directrices de pruebas de la toxicidad reproductiva y ambiental nacionales e internacionales (por ejemplo, de la Organización de Cooperación y Desarrollo Económicos), así como de algunos estudios internacionales de validación de los métodos de prueba. Sin embargo, la posibilidad de que la exposición humana a los contaminantes del medio ambiente (a través de diversas vías) afecte a la función del sistema reproductivo y al desarrollo normal sigue siendo un sector que despierta preocupación a escala mundial.

La reproducción humana normal está regulada por un sistema perfectamente sintonizado de señales coordinadas que dirigen la actividad de numerosas células destinatarias dependientes unas de otras, cuyo resultado es la formación de gametos, su transporte, liberación, fecundación, implantación y gestación y, por último, la formación de descendencia capaz de repetir todo el proceso en condiciones ambientales semejantes o diferentes.

A lo largo de la totalidad del ciclo biológico, todos los aspectos de la función reproductiva dependen de varios sistemas endocrinos de comunicación que utilizan una amplia variedad de hormonas proteicas/peptídicas o esteroídicas, factores de crecimiento y otras moléculas de señalización que influyen en la expresión de los genes de las células destinatarias y/o la síntesis de proteínas. En particular, el desarrollo y la gametogénesis están regulados por una infinidad de señales de intensidad adecuada que se emiten en momentos definidos con precisión. Aunque en estudios recientes en animales se ha demostrado que el desarrollo del feto puede ser más sensible a los efectos de la exposición a las sustancias químicas presentes en el medio ambiente que el sistema adulto, esos efectos podrían no manifestarse hasta la edad adulta. Es fundamental una mayor caracterización de los mecanismos moleculares que regulan los distintos aspectos de la reproducción y el desarrollo normales para comprender la variedad de los mecanismos mediante los cuales las sustancias químicas exógenas pueden perturbar la reproducción y el desarrollo normales.

La función sexual y la fecundidad obedecen a una amplia variedad de funciones que son necesarias para la reproducción y que pueden verse afectadas por la exposición a factores ambientales. Cualquier alteración de la integridad del sistema reproductivo puede afectar a estas funciones. Los modelos de infertilidad notificados varían en todo el mundo, pero alrededor del 10% de las parejas experimentan infertilidad en algún momento durante sus años reproductivos. Los estudios realizados con personas sobre las alteraciones de las funciones sexuales/fecundidad proporcionan el sistema más directo de evaluación del riesgo, pero con frecuencia no se dispone de datos. Para numerosas sustancias químicas presentes en el medio ambiente hay que basarse todavía en información obtenida a partir de modelos con animales experimentales y estudios de laboratorio.

En los estudios *in vivo* con animales para evaluar el riesgo de toxicidad reproductiva se suelen utilizar roedores normales de laboratorio. La evaluación de la fecundidad en los animales machos tiene una sensibilidad limitada como medida de las lesiones reproductivas, porque, a diferencia de las personas, los machos de la mayoría de las especies experimentales producen un volumen de esperma que supera en una medida muy grande el límite necesario para la fecundidad. Los datos histopatológicos de los tejidos reproductivos desempeñan una función importante en la evaluación del riesgo de toxicidad reproductiva en los machos. Se ha demostrado que las sustancias químicas con actividad estrogénica o antiandrogénica pueden tener efectos reproductivos en los machos. Si bien la sensibilidad puede ser diferente, es probable que los mecanismos de acción para estos agentes perturbadores del sistema endocrino sean compatibles o semejantes en todas las especies de mamíferos. Para las hembras, todas las funciones del sistema reproductivo están bajo el control endocrino y pueden verse alteradas por los efectos sobre dicho sistema. Sin embargo, las mediciones aisladas de los cambios hormonales pueden ser indicadores no sensibles de un daño debido a la gran variabilidad de valores normales que se observan en las hembras.

Hay diversos sistemas de prueba *in vitro*, en particular los testículos/ovarios aislados sometidos a perfusión, los cultivos primarios de células gonadales, la investigación de las fracciones subcelulares de diferentes órganos y tipos de células y las técnicas de fecundación *in vitro* que pueden utilizarse en estudios de investigación complementarios de distintos aspectos del sistema reproductivo. Los sistemas de prueba *in vitro* son especialmente útiles para investigar el potencial de toxicidad y para identificar los posibles mecanismos de acción de posibles sustancias tóxicas. Sin embargo, tienen una capacidad limitada para evaluar funciones reproductivas integrativas complejas.

En los últimos años ha sido motivo de creciente preocupación la toxicidad en el desarrollo, definida en su sentido más amplio para incluir todos los efectos adversos en el desarrollo normal, ya sea antes o después del nacimiento. La toxicidad en el desarrollo puede derivarse de la exposición de cualquiera de los padres antes de la concepción, de la exposición del embrión o el feto en el útero o de la exposición de la descendencia después del nacimiento. Los efectos adversos en el desarrollo se pueden detectar en cualquier momento de la vida del organismo. Además de las anomalías estructurales, cabe citar como ejemplos de manifestaciones de la toxicidad en el desarrollo la pérdida del feto, el crecimiento alterado, los defectos funcionales, el brote latente de enfermedades en el adulto, el envejecimiento reproductivo temprano y el acortamiento de la duración de la vida.

En la evaluación de la toxicidad en el desarrollo se han utilizado ampliamente estudios *in vivo* en animales experimentales preñados y su descendencia. El objetivo de las observaciones maternas es evaluar la contribución relativa de su toxicidad a cualquier tipo de toxicidad embrionaria/fetal detectada. Las observaciones en la descendencia incluyen la muerte embrionaria temprana y tardía (resorción), el peso fetal, las malformaciones externas, las anomalías viscerales y esqueléticas y la determinación sexual. La información de antecedentes y los historiales sobre el desarrollo anómalo de animales experimentales son importantes para una interpretación adecuada de dichos estudios de toxicidad. Entre las funciones que se pueden evaluar después del nacimiento figuran el desarrollo neurológico, el comportamiento simple y complejo, la reproducción, la función endocrina, la competencia inmunitaria, el metabolismo xenobiótico y la función fisiológica de distintos sistemas de órganos. Las manifestaciones latentes de la toxicidad pueden ser la carcinogenicidad transplacentaria (neoplasia en la descendencia debido a la exposición materna a agentes químicos durante la preñez) y el acortamiento de la duración de la vida. Para el estudio de la toxicidad en el desarrollo se ha perfeccionado asimismo una amplia variedad de sistemas *in vitro*, que van desde el cultivo de embriones completos, pasando por el cultivo de órganos y tejidos, hasta diversos sistemas de no mamíferos. Las pruebas *in vitro* son útiles en la investigación de los mecanismos del desarrollo normal y anormal para obtener información sobre la relación dosis-respuesta y la toxicidad de órganos específicos, y tal vez como sistemas de investigación para seleccionar o dar prioridad a determinadas sustancias químicas con vistas a nuevos estudios *in vivo*.

Los efectos finales más viables para la evaluación de la toxicidad en el desarrollo humano son las condiciones vitales en el nacimiento (incluida la pérdida embrionaria/fetal), las anomalías congénitas fácilmente identificables, la duración de la gestación, el peso al nacer y la razón de sexos. Los efectos medibles en el desarrollo después del nacimiento incluyen cambios en el crecimiento, el comportamiento y la función de los órganos o sistemas, así como el cáncer. Tanto los efectos prenatales como los posnatales pueden no ser manifiestos hasta bastante después del nacimiento, y algunos pueden no aparecer hasta la edad adulta. Por ejemplo, algunas anomalías congénitas no son observables inmediatamente y sólo ahora se están comenzando a apreciar las secuelas a largo plazo del crecimiento intrauterino retardado. La exposición química durante el desarrollo puede afectar también a la función reproductiva posterior de la descendencia. Por ejemplo, las sustancias químicas pueden dañar las células germinales femeninas en el útero y afectar a la fecundidad de la hembra madura; de igual manera, las células germinales masculinas o células de Sertoli pueden disminuir, pudiendo afectar a la producción de esperma.

En muchos países se han elaborado procedimientos de evaluación del riesgo para la toxicidad reproductiva y en el desarrollo a fin de establecer normas y reglamentar la exposición. En estos procedimientos suele haber componentes de identificación del peligro, relación dosis-respuesta, evaluación de la exposición y caracterización del riesgo. Los protocolos de las pruebas experimentales se basan en gran medida en la identificación de anomalías estructurales y/o carencias funcionales tras la exposición química durante las fases decisivas del ciclo reproductivo. Se deben examinar todas las fuentes disponibles de datos procedentes de animales y de personas para evaluar los efectos tóxicos específicos en la reproducción y el desarrollo. Han mejorado los enfoques para evaluar y resumir los datos relativos a la toxicidad reproductiva. No obstante, con frecuencia se deben formular hipótesis en el proceso de evaluación del riesgo debido a la existencia de lagunas en los conocimientos acerca de los procesos biológicos sobre los que se basan y a las diferencias entre especies. Los métodos y estrategias de las pruebas de evaluación del riesgo se deben perfeccionar continuamente, a medida que se vaya disponiendo de nuevos datos y tecnologías.

2. Recomendaciones

A fin de utilizar estrategias eficaces de control e intervención con objeto de evitar la toxicidad reproductiva y en el desarrollo, se debe establecer una base de conocimientos adecuada. Para mejorar esta base de conocimientos se formulan la recomendaciones siguientes:

1. Establecer y perfeccionar mejores marcadores (moleculares) de los efectos en la reproducción y el desarrollo. Los que pudieran tener una correspondencia humana y animal serían particularmente útiles y ayudarían en la evaluación y el uso de los datos procedentes de animales en la evaluación del riesgo para las personas.

2. Examinar la utilidad de las tecnologías más recientes relacionadas con la expresión de los genes (por ejemplo, conjuntos de genes, proteómica, microscopía de captura por láser) como ayuda para comprender y aclarar los mecanismos subyacentes de la función reproductiva y el desarrollo normales y anormales.

3. Mejorar y perfeccionar métodos para evaluar tanto las fases decisivas de exposición en todo el espectro del desarrollo como las etapas del desarrollo más vulnerables a las manifestaciones de efectos adversos.

4. Mejorar los conocimientos básicos de los mecanismos de la fisiología reproductiva masculina a un nivel comparable con los

conocimientos actuales sobre los mecanismos de la fisiología reproductiva femenina.

5. Promover la aplicación de los conocimientos celulares y moleculares de las funciones de las gónadas y los gametos para mejorar los conocimientos acerca de los efectos toxicológicos en estos tejidos.

6. Buscar y validar modelos de animales para analizar los aspectos toxicológicos de la biología reproductiva, a fin de perfeccionar sistemas adecuados que sean reproducibles, de bajo costo y más fáciles de extrapolar a enfermedades humanas.

7. Mejorar y validar métodos *in vitro* para evaluar mecanismos de una posible toxicidad reproductiva.

8. Promover métodos más exactos y eficaces de medición de la exposición humana a las sustancias químicas presentes en el medio ambiente con una posible toxicidad reproductiva.

9. Mejorar la vigilancia, la recopilación y la armonización de los datos sobre la frecuencia y la distribución geográfica de los defectos congénitos y los trastornos en el desarrollo, prestando particular atención al establecimiento de registros completos.

10. Fomentar las actividades de investigación para identificar mejor las subpoblaciones potencialmente vulnerables a los efectos de los agentes responsables de la toxicidad reproductiva y para caracterizar los factores que contribuyen al aumento de la vulnerabilidad.

11. Habida cuenta de la sensibilidad del organismo durante el desarrollo, prestar mayor atención a los estudios de toxicidad relativos a la exposición durante la gestación o en el período perinatal a una sustancia química o a mezclas de ellas.

12. Utilizar cohortes de nacimientos previamente estudiadas para investigar la incidencia de los resultados reproductivos adversos latentes a lo largo de la vida (las cohortes con datos de exposición durante el embarazo son enormemente importantes).

13. Establecer un sistema armonizado internacional para la terminología y las definiciones en relación con la toxicidad reproductiva y en el desarrollo.